Clinical Neurological Examination and Localization

Vinit Suri

Clinical Neurological Examination and Localization

Springer

Vinit Suri
Department of Neurology
Indraprastha Apollo Hospital
New Delhi, Delhi
India

ISBN 978-981-16-1230-5 ISBN 978-981-16-1228-2 (eBook)
https://doi.org/10.1007/978-981-16-1228-2

This Springer imprint is published by the registered company Springer Nature Singapore Pte Ltd.
The registered company address is: 152 Beach Road, #21-01/04 Gateway East, Singapore 189721, Singapore

Acknowledgments

I would like to thank all my teachers who introduced me to neurology and taught me the art and science of neurological examination and localization which remains extremely relevant even in this era of sophisticated investigations. I am grateful to all my patients who have contributed toward my continued learning and understanding of this complex scientific art of localization. I am also grateful to the wide range of textbooks and scientific literature which helped me in writing this book.

This book is dedicated to my family including my respected late father Shri Virendra Suri, my caring mother Dr Mrs. Satya Suri, my dear wife and my greatest support Dr Neelam Suri, and my loving children Dr Kunal and Dr Kanika who have in their own ways contributed to the completion of this manuscript.

Contents

About the Author

Vinit Suri is one of the most eminent neurologists in India with more than 30 years of experience in the field. He is a graduate of the University College of Medical Sciences, Delhi University, and stood first in the Final MBBS examination with several gold medals to his credit and obtained his D.M. Neurology from G.B. Pant Hospital in 1992. He has been involved in teaching graduate and postgraduate students since the last 30 years and this is something very close to his heart. He is extremely sought after by his students for teaching neurological examination methods and skills of localization in a simple and easy to understand manner.

He has been working at Indraprastha Apollo Hospital, New Delhi, as Senior Consultant Neurologist and Coordinator of the department since 1996 and has been a pioneer in spearheading the Stroke Thrombolysis Program in India.

He has served the Indian Stroke Association as the Secretary, Treasurer, and President and the Delhi Neurological Association as its President.

1 Introduction

Neurological evaluation is similar to solving a complex mathematical equation. It is similar because neurological localization is extremely accurate when components of the equation are selected appropriately. This exercise involves accurate selection of the components of the equation from the history and elicitation of appropriate clinical signs as well as understanding the "neurological language" so as to arrange the components appropriately. An experienced neurologist can take an appropriate though detailed and focused history and conduct an appropriate and focused neurological examination and resulting in localizing the lesion within a few minutes when the inexperienced beginner may not get anywhere even after spending hours.

In this era of sophisticated neurological investigations including MRI, PET MRI, and functional MRI, electrophysiology and genetic and serological markers clinical localization continues to be important and relevant and should not only precede these investigations but also should guide the diagnostic evaluation process.

This book is planned to provide a concise though focused overview of methods of neurological examination enabling a focused clinical approach for localization in patients with neurological disorders.

Important components of the neurological diagnosis include:

1. Site of lesion:
   (a) Central or peripheral nervous system with specific localization site—determined by localization from both history and clinical examination.
2. Etiology of lesion:
   (b) Determined predominantly from the history with clues from:
      I. Onset-acute, subacute, or chronic
      II. Course of the illness-monophasic, relapsing, progressive, or spontaneous improvement
      III. Other comorbidities and family history
      IV. Therapeutic responses and failures

A *Differential Diagnosis* in order of priority is then prepared using the components of the SITE of lesion and ETIOLOGY at that site.

1.1 Basic Neuroanatomy

The nervous system is divided into three important components:

1. Central nervous system
2. Peripheral nervous system
3. Autonomic nervous system (Fig. 1.1)

V. Suri, *Clinical Neurological Examination and Localization*,
https://doi.org/10.1007/978-981-16-1228-2_1

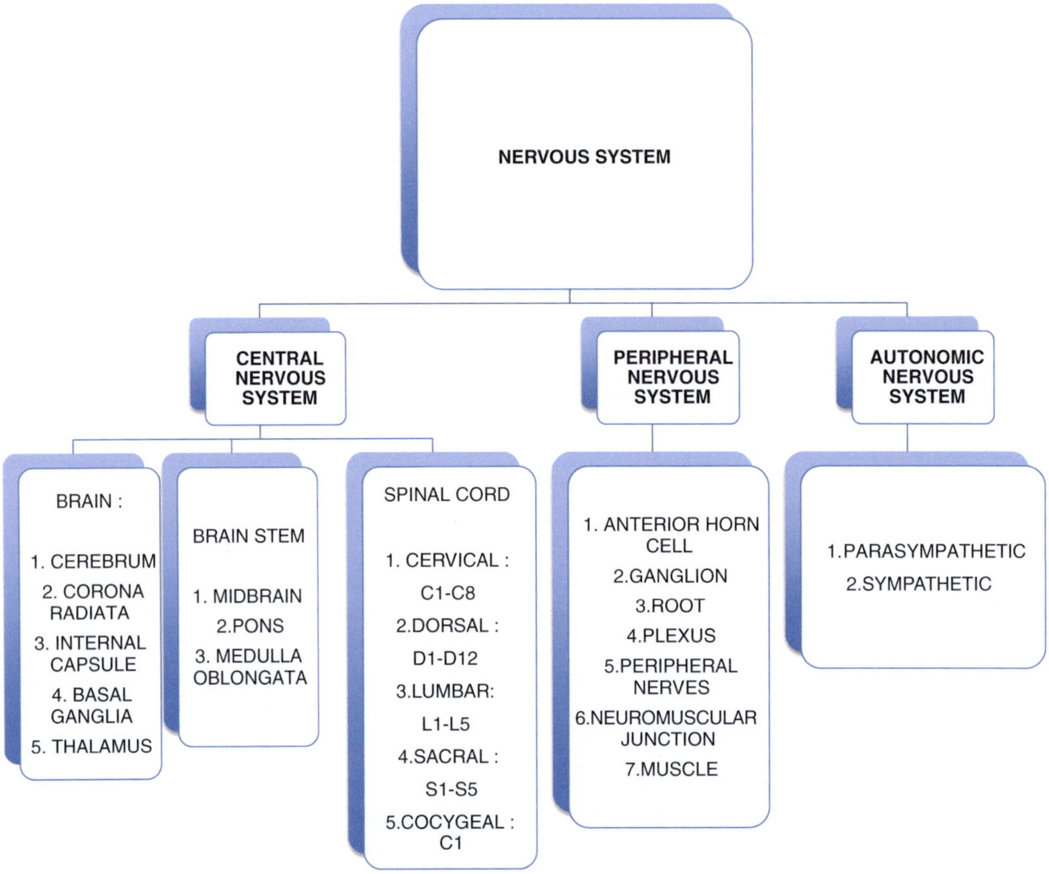

Fig. 1.1 Nervous system—CNS and PNS

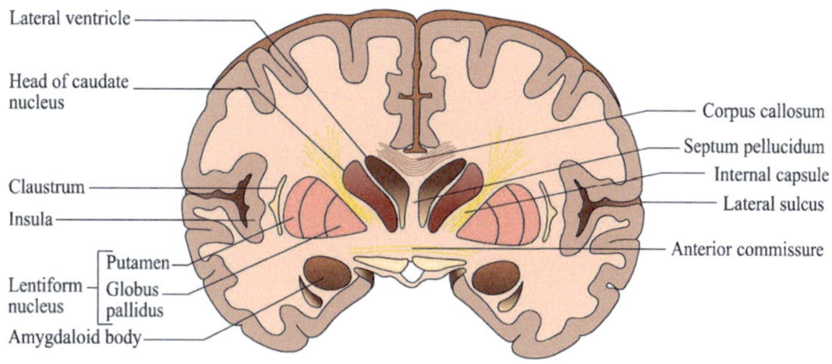
Lateral ventricle
Head of caudate nucleus
Claustrum
Insula
Lentiform nucleus
Putamen
Globus pallidus
Amygdaloid body
Corpus callosum
Septum pellucidum
Internal capsule
Lateral sulcus
Anterior commissure

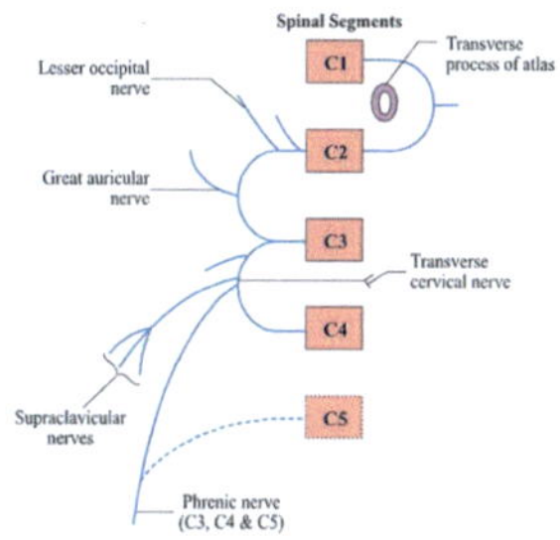
Spinal Segments
C1
C2
C3
C4
C5
Lesser occipital nerve
Great auricular nerve
Transverse process of atlas
Transverse cervical nerve
Supraclavicular nerves
Phrenic nerve (C3, C4 & C5)

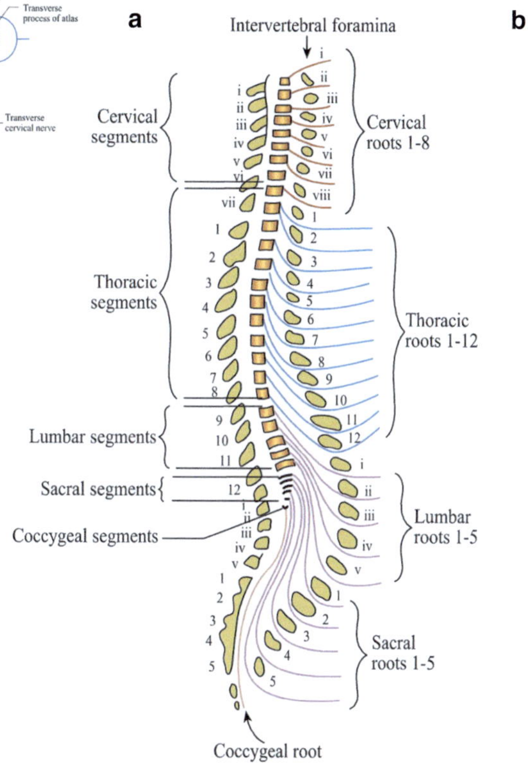
a
b
Intervertebral foramina
Cervical segments
Thoracic segments
Lumbar segments
Sacral segments
Coccygeal segments
Cervical roots 1-8
Thoracic roots 1-12
Lumbar roots 1-5
Sacral roots 1-5
Coccygeal root

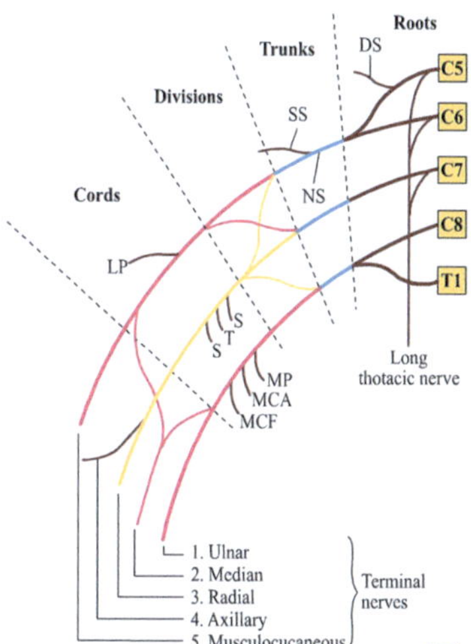
Roots
Trunks
Divisions
Cords
DS
SS
NS
LP
S
T
S
MP
MCA
MCF
C5
C6
C7
C8
T1
Long thotacic nerve
1. Ulnar
2. Median
3. Radial
4. Axillary
5. Musculocucaneous
Terminal nerves

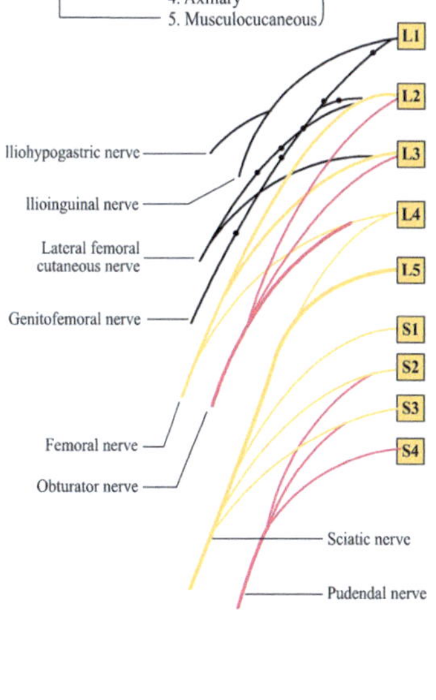
L1
L2
L3
L4
L5
S1
S2
S3
S4
Iliohypogastric nerve
Ilioinguinal nerve
Lateral femoral cutaneous nerve
Genitofemoral nerve
Femoral nerve
Obturator nerve
Sciatic nerve
Pudendal nerve

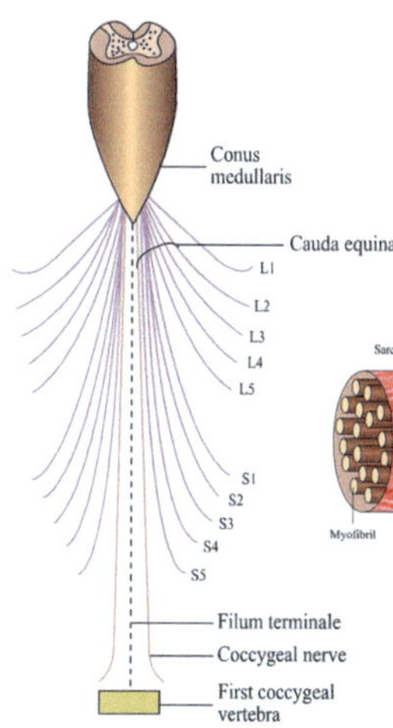
Conus medullaris
Cauda equina
L1
L2
L3
L4
L5
S1
S2
S3
S4
S5
Filum terminale
Coccygeal nerve
First coccygeal vertebra

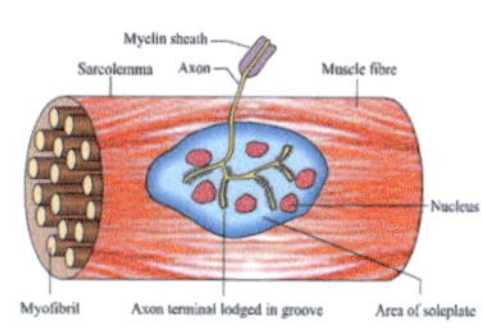
Myelin sheath
Sarcolemma
Axon
Muscle fibre
Nucleus
Myofibril
Axon terminal lodged in groove
Area of soleplate

2 The Neurological History

History is the most important part of the neurological evaluation and a skillfully obtained history should be able to give a fair idea about the diagnosis regarding both the *site* and the *etiology* of the neurological illness. The experienced neurologist will listen attentively to the history narrated by the patient, remaining alert to subtle clues, question the patient for additional information, and then place the details into a correct context and organize the facts into a coherent framework to lead toward the diagnosis.

2.1 Components

2.1.1 Demographics

- Name
- Age
- Sex
- Occupation/education level
- Handedness (left hemisphere is dominant in 99% of right handed individuals and in 60–70% of left handed or ambidextrous individuals)
- Reliability of history
- Informant

2.1.2 History of Present Illness

1. The patient should be requested to inform the problems from the beginning and in order of evolution of *symptoms*. The chief complaint and the history of present illness should be documented preferably in the patient's own words. Patients should be encouraged to explain the symptoms rather than using terminology, e.g., "blackout" which could mean vision loss or pre-syncopal greying of consciousness or loss of consciousness. Symptoms should be corroborated from accompanying eye witnesses whenever possible and especially if the patient has had altered sensorium, memory issues or loss of insight.
2. Particular emphasis should be laid to identify the *course* of each important neurological symptom:
   (a) Onset: Instantaneous, abrupt onset, or insidious onset
   (b) Course: Monophasic, progressive, relapsing, spontaneous remission, or recovery with treatment
3. *Detailed* evaluation of each symptom should be performed so as to obtain information about its source of origin and mode of onset.

2.1.2.1 Specific Questions to be Enquired in Certain Common Neurological Symptoms

Motor Weakness

1. Distribution of weakness: Distal, proximal, selective muscle groups, hemiplegia,

V. Suri, *Clinical Neurological Examination and Localization*,
https://doi.org/10.1007/978-981-16-1228-2_2

paraplegia or quadriplegia, radicular, or nerve distribution.

2. Accompanying wasting or hypertrophy (prominent and early wasting is suggestive of a LMN lesion and pseudohypertrophy is usually seen in muscular dystrophies).
3. Accompanying fasciculations (seen commonly in anterior horn cell disease), or trophic changes.
4. Subjective feeling of looseness (hypotonia) or stiffness
(spasticity/rigidity) of limbs.
5. Important clues to subjective versus definite motor weakness.
   (a) Difficulty in buttoning–unbuttoning or opening jar would indicate definite distal upper limb weakness.
   (b) Difficulty in combing hair or applying soap on scalp would indicate definite proximal upper limb weakness.
   (c) Slipping of footwear from feet (with awareness would be suggestive of definite weakness of small muscles of foot and slippage without awareness would be suggestive of posterior column loss in foot. Getting footwear into bed without awareness would indicate severe posterior column loss of sensation in the foot).
6. True fatigability—Marked worsening following repetitive motor acts is usually suggestive of neuromuscular junction pathology. e.g., myasthenia gravis. Mild nonspecific fatigability, however, will occur in most weak muscles from any cause.

Headache

- Paroxysmal or non-paroxysmal: (paroxysmal is often a feature of vascular headaches and continuous headache is often a feature in patients with muscle contraction cephalgia or in patients with secondary headaches.)
- Character: Whether headache is throbbing, non-throbbing, "cap on head" like feel, itching, burning or something moving over scalp (Throbbing headache is usually seen in patients with migraine or other vascular causes and non-throbbing dull stretching pain maybe indicative of a muscle contraction cephalgia).
- Distribution: Whether the headache is localized or holocranial or headache spreading to craniofascial distribution or entire hemisensory distribution of one side of the body.
- Aggravating and relieving factors and periodicity
- (Migraine pain is usually aggravated with exposure to bright sunlight, outdoor travel, sleep deprivation, fasting, strong odors, and certain dietary products, e.g., cheese, alcohol, or chocolates whereas muscle contraction headache is usually aggravated with emotional stress). Secondary headaches from raised intracranial pressure may worsen with coughing, sneezing, or straining.
- Accompanying symptoms, e.g., nausea, vomiting, visual blurring, photophobia, phonophobia, conjunctival congestion, lacrimation, or nasal block (Accompanying photophobia and phonophobia is usually seen in patients with migraine and ipsilateral nasal block with ipsilateral conjunctival congestion and lacrimation is seen in patients with cluster headache).
- Accompanying neurological symptoms, e.g., diplopia, motor weakness or visual acuity or field loss are usually indicative of secondary headaches.

Seizure

- Any premonitory remembered symptoms (aura or pre-syncopal greying).
- Ictal description of minor or major motor movements, automatisms, duration of loss of awareness and responsiveness, Ictal tongue bite, incontinence or injury, and duration of the episode.
- Post-ictal symptoms (headache, confusion, excessive sleep, behavior abnormalities, and duration of post-ictal symptoms till complete recovery.
- Periodicity.
- Are all the seizures similar or are there different types of seizures.

- Treatment details and response to various drug regimes.
- Family history of seizures and development history of the patient.
- Differentiate from a syncope by enquiring about any presyncopal greying of consciousness at onset, any aggravating vagal stimulating event precipitating the event, profuse sweating and/or cold limbs, pale fascies, ictal injury over face or head and abrupt offset on attaining a horizontal posture with no post-episodic confusion (unless the fall resulted in a component of brain contusion).

Dizziness

- Differentiate various symptoms—Vertigo—definite external whirling with or without nausea and vomiting (involvement of vestibulo-cerebellar pathway).
- Dizziness—Vague, inner sway without definite external whirling (cervicogenic, muscle contraction cephalgia).
- Syncope or pre-syncopal greying—Feeling of passing out or losing consciousness with greying of consciousness.
- Unsteadiness—Imbalance and reeling while walking (involvement of cerebellar pathway).
- Any aggravation by head movement or body posture.
- Accompanying tinnitus, hearing loss, numbness, acral weakness, or unsteadiness.
- Frequency and duration of symptoms and periodicity.

Numbness

- Differentiate between tingling (positive sensation) or numbness (negative sensation).
- Distribution: For example, Glove and stocking distribution (peripheral neuropathy), Cranial nerve distribution, e.g., 5th cranial nerve, Nerve distribution, e.g., Median nerve or Radicular distribution, e.g., C5 root.
- Aggravating factors, e.g., aggravation particularly on attempted sleep is suggestive of restless leg syndrome and aggravation with coughing, sneezing, or straining maybe suggestive of a compressive radiculopathy.
- Any claudication symptoms, i.e., aggravation by time dependent standing or length dependent walking (indicative of peripheral vascular disease or spinal canal stenosis).

Diplopia

- Uniocular (ophthalmic cause) or binocular (neurogenic cause).
- Horizontally separated images (6th nerve palsy) or vertically separated images (3rd or 4th nerve palsy).
- Identify which gaze causes maximum separation of the two images (right, left or superior, inferior).
- True fatigability of diplopia with near resolution after eye closure or sleep (e.g., myasthenia gravis).

Memory Loss

- Subjective or noticed by others
- Duration and course
- Identify the quantum of disability, e.g., continuing with all activities including job or significant disability requiring assistance.
- Any depressive or anxiety symptoms, any past history of stroke.
- Any family history of dementia or Alzheimer's disease.
- Any addictions or medication use that may contribute to memory impairment.

2.2 Specific Questions

Certain pertinent questions regarding specific neurological symptoms are enquired into since these symptoms provide important insights regarding the sites of involvement of the neural axis.

- Bowel or bladder disturbances (enquire about bladder sensation, hesitancy, or urgency-precipitancy, incontinence—with or without awareness. Also, enquire regarding change of bowel habit, e.g., constipation or fecal incontinence).
- Sexual disturbances.
- Any swelling/bony deformity or growth/areas of tenderness.
- Birth marks (café au lait spots, hemangioma), acquired skin lesions (hypopigmentation and hypoanesthetic areas in Hansen's disease).

2.3 Negative History

Important and focused negative histories relevant to the case should be enquired into:

- Arthralgia's—small or large joints or both
- Oral ulcers/genital ulcers (SLE, Behchet's)
- Rashes
- Constitutional symptoms—fatigue, weight loss, anorexia
- Dryness of mouth, eyes (Sjogren's syndrome)
- Symptoms pertaining to individual cranial nerves
- Tremulousness of limbs
- Gait abnormality
- Hypoesthetic and differentially pigmented single or multiple lesions, e.g., Hansen's disease

2.4 Past Medical History

1. Other comorbities, e.g., hypertension, hypothyroidism, diabetes, coronary artery disease, peripheral vascular disease or vasculitis with reference to duration, and details of treatment taken since certain neurological disorders maybe related to these systemic disorders.
   (a) Assess details of medication used since some symptoms may be related to drug-related adverse effects.
2. Past history of any neurological disorder, e.g., TIA in stroke patients, recurrent neurological deficit in multiple sclerosis.
3. Assess details of major past medical illnesses and past surgical history.

2.5 Family History

Detailed family history is important since many neurological disorders have a genetic basis. A family tree maybe drawn with for 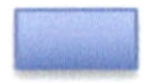 males and 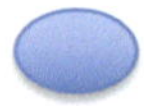 for females and an arrow indicating the patient in question (Fig. 2.1).

- Vertical transmission in generations is suggestive of an autosomal dominant inheritance pattern.
- Horizontal transmission in the same generation is suggestive of an autosomal recessive inheritance pattern.
- Sex-linked inheritance is indicated when only males are involved and females are carriers.
- Assess relationship between parents, especially regarding consanguinity.
- Assess the ethnic background since certain disorders maybe more often seen in certain ethnic groups.

2.6 Social History

It is important to assess social history regarding:

- Education level of the patient.
- Occupation—assess the exact nature of work with special reference to exposure to any neurotoxins.
- Married/never married/divorced.
- Ethanol, tobacco chewing, smoking history, or any substance abuse.
- Diet—vegetarian diet or inflammatory bowel disease may induce vitamin B12 deficiency-related disorders.

2.7 Neurological Examination

2.7.1 Format

Neurological Examination is conducted and recorded in a standard *format*.

1. Mental state and *Higher mental functions*
   (a) Initial screen

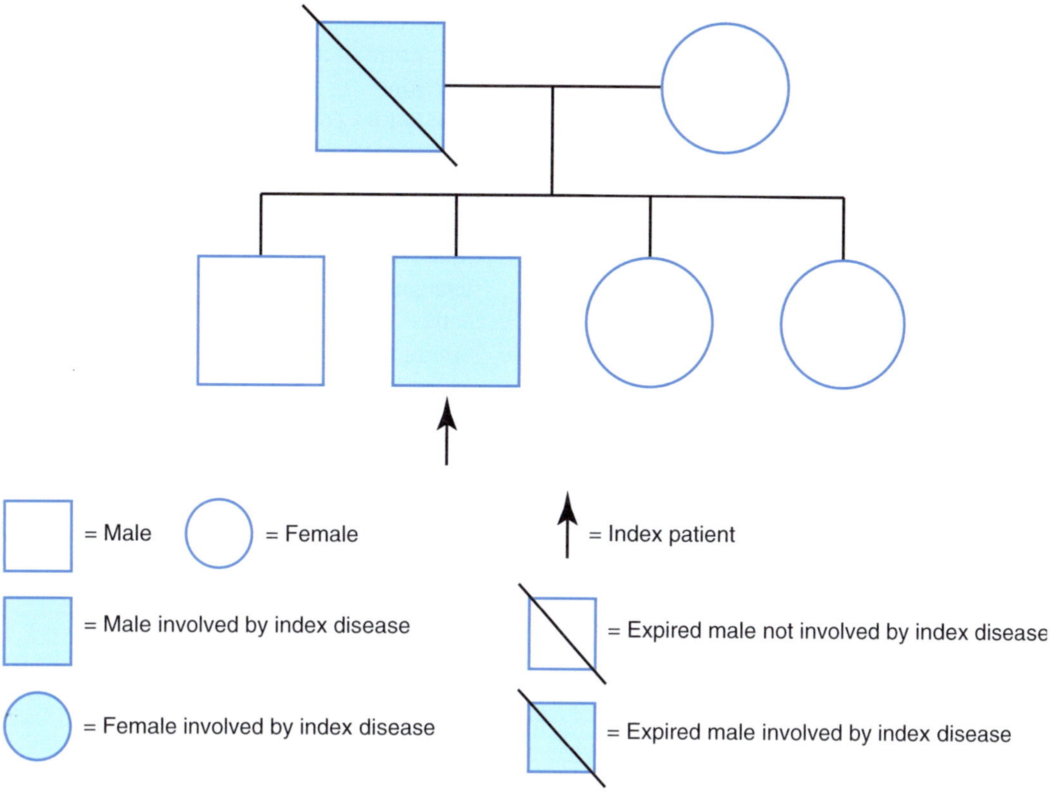

Fig. 2.1 Family tree

   (b) Lobar function assessment when indicated
2. Speech
   (a) Language disorders—Aphasia
   (b) Enunciation disorders—Dysarthria
   (c) Volume of speech disorders—Dysphonia
3. Cranial nerves 1–12
4. Motor system evaluation
   (a) Inspection—bulk, involuntary movements
   (b) Tone
   (c) Motor power
5. Sensory system evaluation
   (a) Exteroceptive—pain, temperature
   (b) Proprioceptive—touch, vibration, joint position
   (c) Cortical sensations—astereognosis, graphasthesia, two point discrimination, tactile localization, sensory inattention
6. Reflexes—superficial and deep tendon reflexes
7. Coordination and cerebellar evaluation
8. Posture, Stance, and Gait
9. Skull, Spine, Peripheral nerves and Neuro cutaneous markers.
10. Autonomic nervous system

2.8 The Neurological Kit

The neurological examination requires certain instruments, which should be available with the evaluator at all times as a prepared handy to use kit.

- Percussion hammer
- Torch or penlight
- Ophthalmoscope
- Tuning fork 128 hz—for testing vibration
- Tuning fork 512 hz—for testing Rinne and Weber
- Two point discriminator
- Sterile pin, rolling pin-wheel for testing pain
- Test tubes—to check temperature sensation (fill with water 30° and 47° C)
- Cotton—wisp for testing touch and corneal reflex
- Smell bottles containing—vanilla, chocolate, coffee, and perfume for evaluating olfaction
- Taste bottles containing—sugar, salt, vinegar, neem powder or chloroquine powder, and sterile cotton buds
- Measuring tape
- Coins, rubber band, pen—to be used for stereognosis
- Stethoscope
- Pinhole with reading charts and color charts

3 Higher Mental Function

3.1 Higher Mental Function

Higher mental function assessment is the most tedious aspect of the neurological examination, especially when the patient has significant disability and it may take an extremely long time to conduct this part of the examination due to delayed responses, poor comprehension, and difficulty in completing the tasks by the patient.

(A) Most patients are initially evaluated by a *limited screening test for higher mental functions*.
(B) In select patients with disability on the screening testing, *detailed lobar function* testing is conducted to localize the clinical deficits.

Before initiating the higher mental function testing explain to the patient that a simple mental evaluation will be conducted and that these questions may seem to be very basic and that the patient should not be annoyed because of the simplicity of some of the questions (most patients get upset as to why these basic and simple questions are being asked!!!).

3.2 Screening Tests of Higher Mental Function

1. Attention and vigilance
2. Orientation
3. Calculation
4. Visuo-spatial tests
5. Abstract thinking
6. Judgement
7. Apraxia and Agnosias
8. Appearance, behavior, mood, and perceptual disturbances

3.2.1 Attention Span and Vigilance

Attention span is the duration the patient can focus on a task without getting distracted.

Vigilance is a sustained maintenance of attention over a period of time and is measured by the focus of the patient during the elicitation of the entire history and examination.

V. Suri, *Clinical Neurological Examination and Localization*,
https://doi.org/10.1007/978-981-16-1228-2_3

Substrate Attention span is regulated by a polysynaptic pathway between the cerebral cortex, cortical alerting pathways to the mesencephalic reticular formation projecting through the thalamus.

Attention is subdivided into:

(a) Active
- Voluntarily generated and directed.
- Mediated by superior parietal lobule and dorsal prefrontal cortex.

(b) Passive
- Involuntarily trigged by external stimulation and basic drives.
- Generated more in nondominant hemisphere.
- Mediated by inferior parietal lobule and posterior portion of superior temporal gyrus.

Clinical Tests

(i) Digit span—Ask the patient to repeat 3–4 digit numbers and then increase the number of digits (numbers should not be in a sequence or pattern but should be randomly placed).

Normal response—Repetition of a 7-digit number forward.

Ask the patient to repeat the digits backward or spell the word "WORLD" backward.

Normal—5 digit backward.

(ii) Cross out all the letters "A" in a sheet with randomly written letters and notice missed out letters or wrong letters being marked.

Clinical Relevance

(i) Attention span deficit occurs with disruption of the polysynaptic corticoreticular pathway, especially frontal lobe dysfunction predominantly of the nondominant hemisphere.

(ii) Attention span is commonly impaired in toxic and metabolic encephalopathies.

(iii) Defective attention can affect the responses to most of the subsequently tested higher mental function tests and further tests should be modified proportionately to the attention span.

3.2.2 Orientation

Orientation is evaluated for:

(i) TIME—Time (normal response is the ability to inform the correct time up to half an hour–less or more), day, date, month, and year.

(ii) PLACE—Floor, hospital, locality, city, state, country.

(iii) PERSON—Enquire about relatives, doctors, nurses, and whether the patient can identify them correctly.

(iv) INSIGHT—Awareness of the medical situation and disabilities.

3.2.3 Memory

Human memory can be subdivided into a number of subtypes:

1. Immediate recall
2. Recent memory (short term)
3. Remote memory (long term)

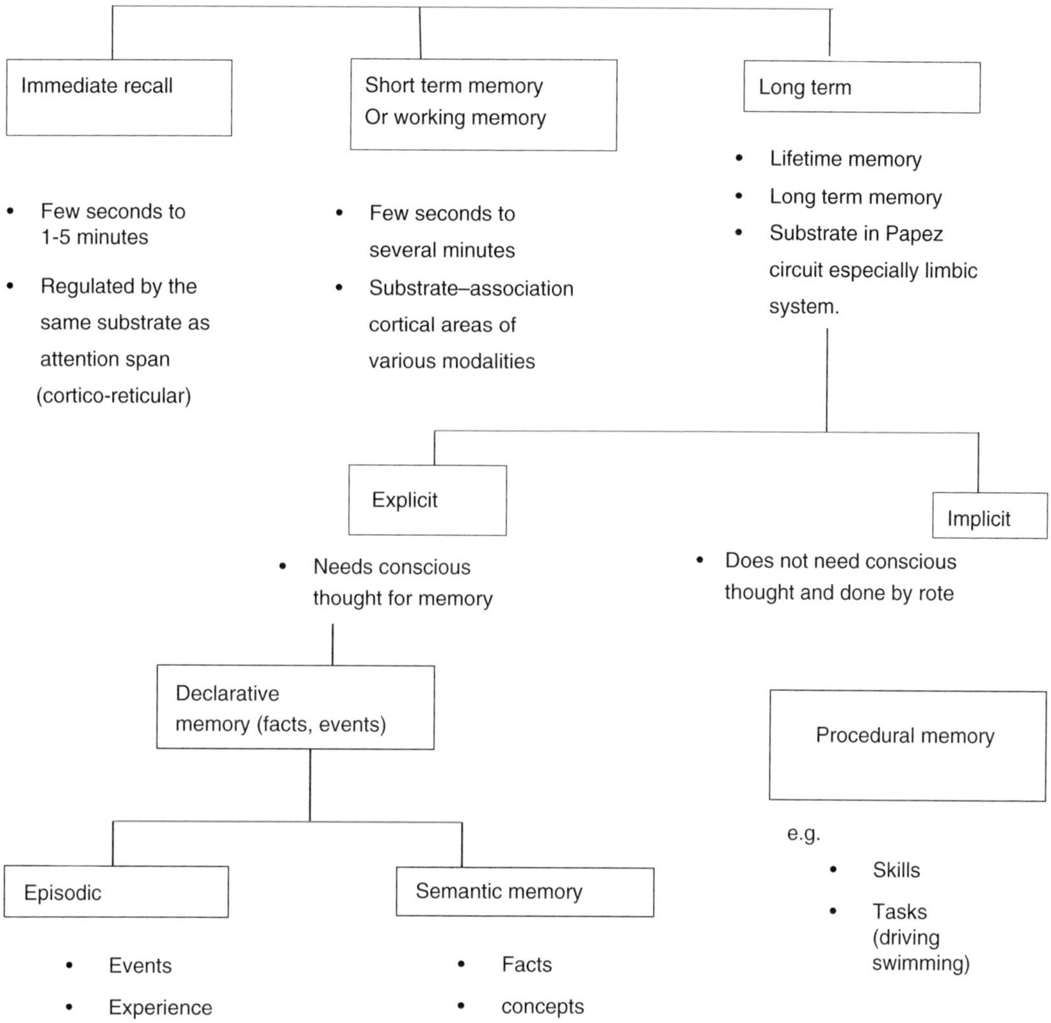

Immediate Recall

- Memory of few seconds to one minute.
- Substrate is similar to "Attention span, i.e., cortico-reticular polysynaptic pathway.

Test:

(i) Ask the patient to repeat an address, or a sentence.
(ii) Forward and backward digit span (Normal—Forward digit span >7 and backward digit span >5).

Short-Term Memory

- Memory of a few seconds to few minutes.
- Substrate is in the various association cortices of the particular modality of memory.

E.g., Memory for faces—lingual gyri.
Tactile memory—somatosensory area.

- Visual memory is represented in the nondominant hemisphere and Verbal memory is represented in the dominant hemisphere.

Test:

(i) Verbal memory (dominant hemisphere) gives 5 unrelated words (e.g., coin, fly, wood, happiness, and apple) and ask the patient to memorize them and that he/she will be asked to recall these 5 items later.
  - Note the number of attempts to remember all 5 words.
  - Ask the patient to repeat the words after 4–5 min (meanwhile distract the patient by conducting some other tests).

(ii) Visual memory (nondominant hemisphere).
Show 5 objects and place them around the patient, e.g., watch below pillow, and pen in your pocket.
Ask the patient to remember all the 5 objects and where they are placed and note the number of attempts needed to memorize the 5 objects.
Ask the names of the 5 objects and where they are hidden after 5 min.

(iii) Ask the patient what he/she had in the last meal.

Long-Term Memory

Substrate: Papez circuit (limbic system)—which includes the hippocampus, fornix, mammillary bodies, mammillothalamic tract, anterior and dorsomedial thalamic nucleus, cingulate gyrus, and cingulum.

Test:

(i) Fund of information: Ask about previous events, facts, and concepts.
For example, when did India get independence, who was the first president of India?

(ii) Personal information: Where and when were you married?
Where and when did you get your college/school degree?

(iii) Episodic memory: is evaluated for both verbal and visual aspects:
verbal—e.g., what all did u eat in the last meal?
Visual—e.g., describe the location of your house and the buildings around your house?

(iv) Semantic memory: is evaluated for both verbal and visual aspects.
verbal—e.g., naming household objects, months of the year, countries starting with letter A.
visual—recognizing famous persons from their photographs.

(v) Working memory: impaired working memory is a part of impaired executive function and is usually abnormal in patients with lesions of the prefrontal cortex, e.g., appropriate planning of a dinner party for 10 persons by a housewife or planning a conference meeting of the various office bearers by an office executive.

(vi) Procedural memory: ability to use previously learned skills, e.g., ability to use a screw driver or a shovel or a mobile phone. Abnormality is seen with lesions of the supplementary motor area (frontal lobe).

3.2.4 Calculation

Substrate: Impairment of calculations is seen in lesions involving the dominant parietal lobe, especially the angular gyrus.

Tests:

(i) Serial 100-7 (serially subtract 7 from 100 and then again from the number obtained) or simpler evaluations by serial 100 minus 3.

(ii) Doubling numbers, e.g., ask the patient to keep doubling the number, e.g., 3,6 12, 24 … till error occurs.

(iii) Simple calculations—How much is $3 + 3 = 6$?

3.2.5 Abstract Thinking and Judgment

3.2.5.1 Abstract Thinking

The ability to think abstractly is an important part of the higher mental function testing.

Tests:

(i) Narrate proverbs and ask the patient what it means. Look for abnormal concrete thinking, e.g., Grass is greener on the other side of the fence.

Normal response—"It appears other people are in a better situation than us."

Abnormal response—"The color of grass is greener on the other side of the fence."

(ii) Assess ability to identify and rationalize similarities and differences—e.g., spot the odd man out among apple banana and tomato and why? Or bicycle, car, and airplane and why?

Substrate: Abstract thinking impairment can occur with many lesions resulting in cortical dysfunction, but is commonly seen in patients with Frontal lobe disorders.

3.2.5.2 Judgment

This tests for judgmental power of the patient in certain situations and is controlled by a high level of organized mental functioning including memory, planning, and multitasking.

Tests: What will you do if there is a fire in the room?

Normal response—"call for fire ambulance or call out neighbors for help or try to put it out by water."

Abnormal response—"Will call my son in Canada."

Substrate: Impairment can occur with many lesions but is commonly seen in lesions involving orbito-frontal lobe.

3.2.6 Visuospatial Tests

Impairment of visuospatial abilities and impairment of constructional abilities should be evaluated as an important aspect of higher mental function testing.

Test:

(i) Ask the patient to draw a clock with a particular time, e.g., 3:30. Abnormal—wrong numbers, wrong hand size, or position
   - Hemineglect

(ii) Ask the patient to copy:
   - A star
   - 2-Dimensional square

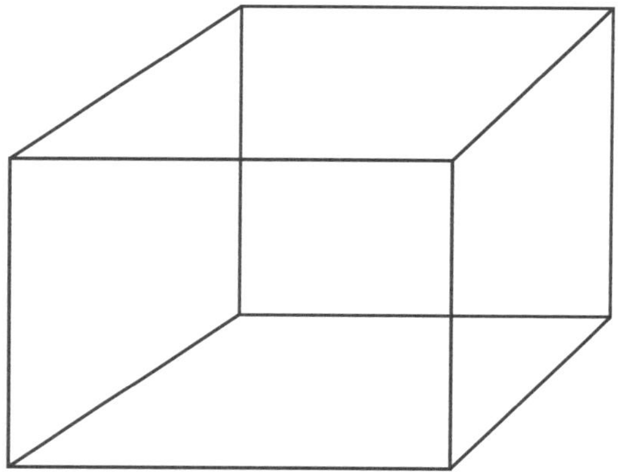

Fig 3.1 Copy a square

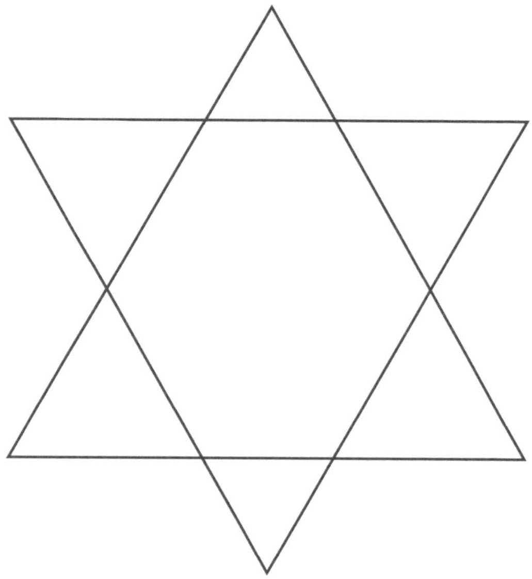

Fig 3.2 Copy a star

Substrate: Visuospatial abnormalities are seen in patients with Frontal lobe or Parietal lobe dysfunction (Figs. 3.1 and 3.2).

3.2.7 Apraxia

Apraxia is defined as the inability to carry out a previously learnt motor act in the absence of any motor weakness, sensory loss, or other deficits involving the involved part.

1. Limb kinetic apraxia

   Difficulty in carrying out fine motor acts with a resemblance to clumsiness. It occurs due to mild lesions involving the corticospinal tract (lesion of primary cortex area—precentral gyrus) but not severe enough to cause detectable weakness.

2. Ideomotor (motor) apraxia

   Patient is unable to perform motor acts. For example, salute, wave goodbye, snap the fingers, stand like a boxer. These patients are also unable to imitate motor acts demonstrated by the examiner.

   Occurs due to lesions of dominant parietal lobe or frontal lobe.

   Test:

   (i) Ask the patient to copy your hand movements, e.g., make *a fist, tap it on the table with thumb upward then place your* palm on the table.

   (ii) Pantomime to perform acts like lighting a cigarette, brushing your teeth clearly and carefully demonstrating all the steps involved in the process (observe for planning each aspect of the act and its execution).

3. Ideational (conceptual) apraxia

   Patient is able to carry out individual components of a complex motor act but cannot perform the entire sequence properly and have impaired ability to plan an act that requires several steps, e.g., lift the pen, open the cap, pull out one sheet of paper, write your name on the paper, and close the pen and put the pen back in your pocket.

   - Caused by damage to dominant parietal lobe.

4. Buccofacial or oral apraxia

   Patient is unable to execute complex acts involving lips, mouth, and face, e.g., whistling, coughing, pressing lips, or blowing out a flame in the absence of any weakness of facial muscles.

   - Maybe seen in the parietal lobe or frontal lobe dysfunction of either lobe.

5. Constructional apraxia

   Patient has inability to copy geometric forms of any complexity due to loss of visuospatial skills, e.g., 3-dimensional square.

   - Seen in nondominant parietal lobe lesion.

6. Dressing apraxia

   Patient loses the ability to wear clothing correctly and appropriately with a tendency to mix buttons or wearing a shirt with only one arm in the sleeve or in the neck area. Can evaluate by pulling one arm sleeve of the shirt inside out and handing over the shirt to the patient to wear it.

   Seen commonly in nondominant parietal lobe lesions.

3.2.8 Agnosia

Agnosia is the inability to recognize a sensory stimulus, e.g., visual, tactile, or auditory even though the sensory stimulus is perceived. Agnosia's occur when there is interference of transfer of information from primary sensory cortical area to the language areas. Agnosia occurs in the absence of any impairment of cognition, attention, or loss of sensory modality and is usually specific to the given sensory modality.

Type of Agnosia	Clinical impairment	Site of lesion
Visual agnosia	Inability to recognize objects visually with no impairment of vision	Cortical blindness occurs from lesions of the primary vision area 17, visual agnosia occurs from lesions anterior to it, i.e., posterior occipital and temporal
Auditory agnosia	Inability to recognize familiar sounds, words with intact hearing	Bilateral or dominant anterior superior temporal region
Tactile agnosia	Inability to recognize objects by touch and feel without any sensory loss in the hand (though can feel the texture and weight)	Dominant parietal lobe lesion
Autopagnosia	Inability to recognize and name body parts (body image agnosia)	Dominant parietal lobe
Finger agnosia	Inability to recognize fingers (autopagnosia involving fingers)	Dominant inferior parietal lobe

Time agnosia	Inability to be aware of time sense without disorientation to other modalities	Dominant temporal lobe
Prosopagnosia	Inability to recognize familiar faces (may recognize the person by sound)	Lesion of Fusiform gyrus or bilateral lesions of occipitotemporal lobes dominant
Simultagnosia	Ability to only perceive and concentrate on one object at a time but not the entire picture	Bilateral lesions of the junction of temporal to occipital lobe
Color agnosia	Cannot name the color though is not color blind and can perceive the color and match it with other similar colored objects (also called color anomia)	Dominant occipital lobe

3.2.9 Appearance, Behavior, Mood, Delusions, and Hallucinations

(i) Check whether the patient is appropriately *dressed* or is there self-neglect or incorrect placement of buttons or whether the patient is wearing unmatched clothes (maybe seen in dressing apraxia, frontal lobe dysfunction, depression, or schizophrenia).
(ii) Assess whether patient has normal *mood*, is anxious, or depressed or manic.
(iii) Check for the presence of *perceptual* disturbances:

Delusions—firmly held, wrong belief.

Hallucinations—perception of sensory modality in the absence of a stimulus.

These perceptual disturbances are commonly seen in psychiatric disorders and may occur in patients with encephalopathies or temporal lobe lesions.

3.3 Specific Lobar Function

Detailed lobar function testing is conducted when the initial screen test of higher function testing indicates an abnormality (Figs. 3.3, 3.4, 3.5, 3.6, 3.7, 3.8, 3.9 and 3.10).

3.4 Frontal Lobe

Frontal lobe is the largest of all the 4 lobes and is separated posteriorly from the Parietal lobe by the Central sulcus and inferiorly from the Temporal lobe by the Sylvian fissure (Figs. 3.11, 3.12 and 3.13).

Important Brodmann areas in the Frontal lobe include:

- 4=primary motor cortex
- 6=premotor cortex and supplementary motor cortex
- 8=frontal eye field
- 46, 9=dorsolateral prefrontal cortex
- 10=anterior prefrontal cortex
- 44=Brocas
- 43=primary gustatory
- 11, 12=orbitofrontal

The frontal lobe is divided into 6 important functional zones and functional testing is conducted accordingly.

1. Primary motor cortex (precentral gyrus—Brodmann area 4)
2. Premotor area
3. Frontal eye field area (area 8)
4. Supplementary motor area (area 6)
5. Speech (dominant lobe, area 44)
6. Prefrontal area (include 9, 10, 11, 12, 32, 45, 47)—lies anterior to areas 6 and 8 and is subdivided into:
   (a) Dorsolateral prefrontal region
   (b) Medial prefrontal region
   (c) Orbitofrontal region

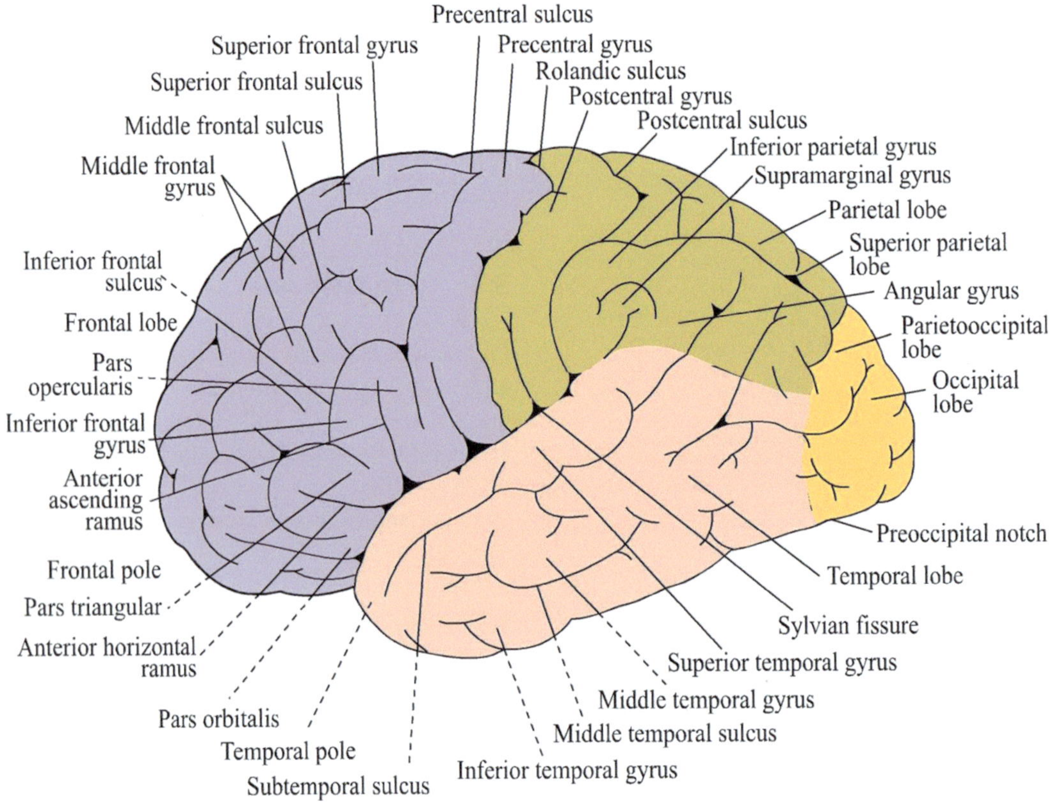

Fig 3.3 Supero lateral surface-cortical areas

3.4.1 Functions and Tests According to Functional Regions of Frontal Lobe

3.4.1.1 Primary Motor Cortex (Area 4)

Lesions result in contralateral hemiplegia(non-dense) with extensor plantar response due to involvement of corticospinal and corticobulbar tracts.

3.4.2 Premotor Area

Lies squeezed between and anterior to precentral gyrus and posterior to area 6.

1. Involved in planning and execution of movement.
2. Tests for kinetic melodies.

(a) Motor Luria test (fist-edge—palm test). Patient is asked to perform sequential movements by placing firstly the fist on the table, and then placing the edge of the palm on the table and then the hand on the table with palm upward and is asked to repeat the movement repeatedly.

(b) Ring-fist test—patient is asked to repeatedly and alternatively make a fist and ring (using thumb and index finger) with either hand. Abnormal response would result in repeated errors with either multiple rings only or multiple fists only without a smooth alternate switch between fist and ring.

(c) Luria graphic test—patient should copy a diagram with alternating sequence, e.g., triangle and square (Fig. 3.14).

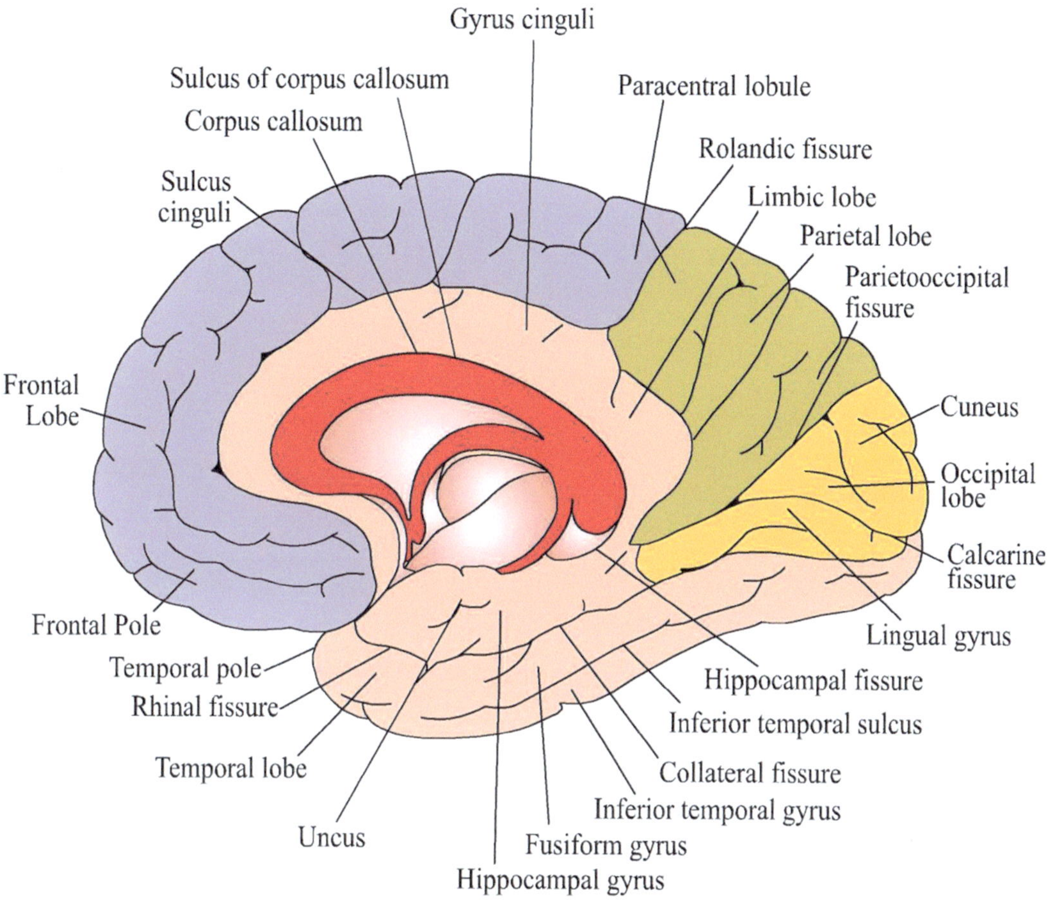

Fig 3.4 Mesial surface-cortical areas

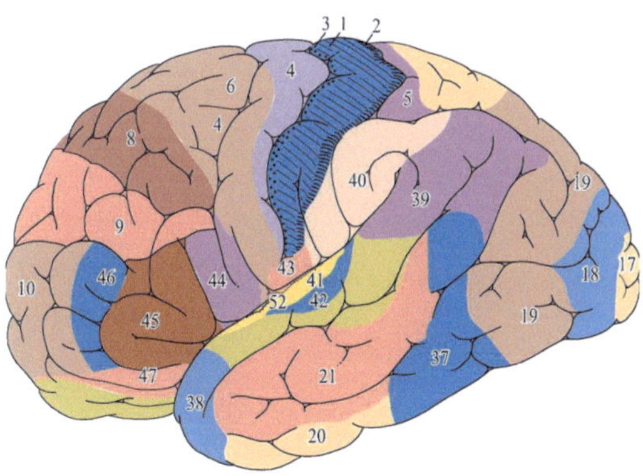

Fig 3.5 Broadman areas of superolateral surface

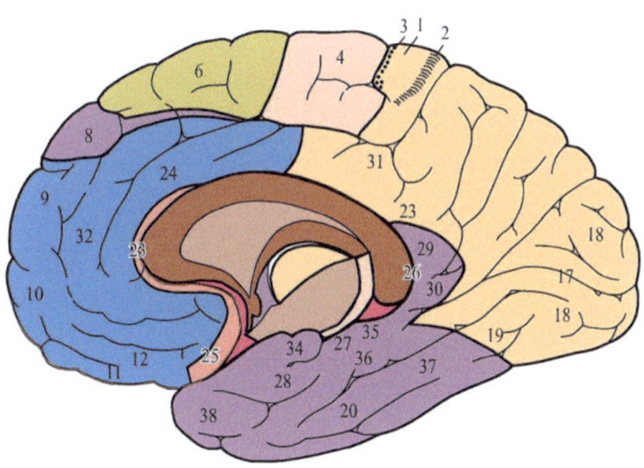

Fig 3.6 Broadman areas of mesial surface

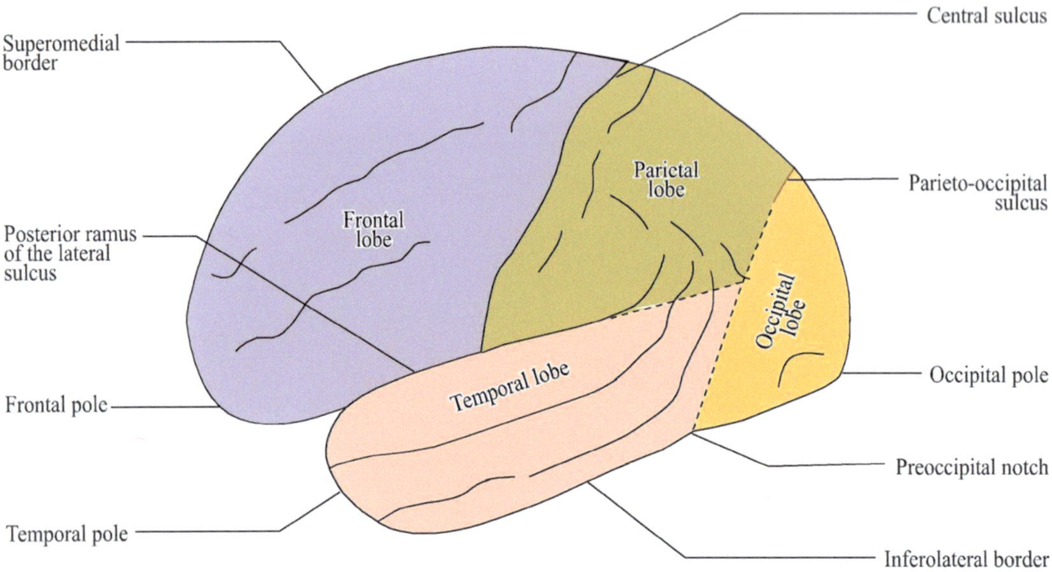

Fig 3.7 Lobes

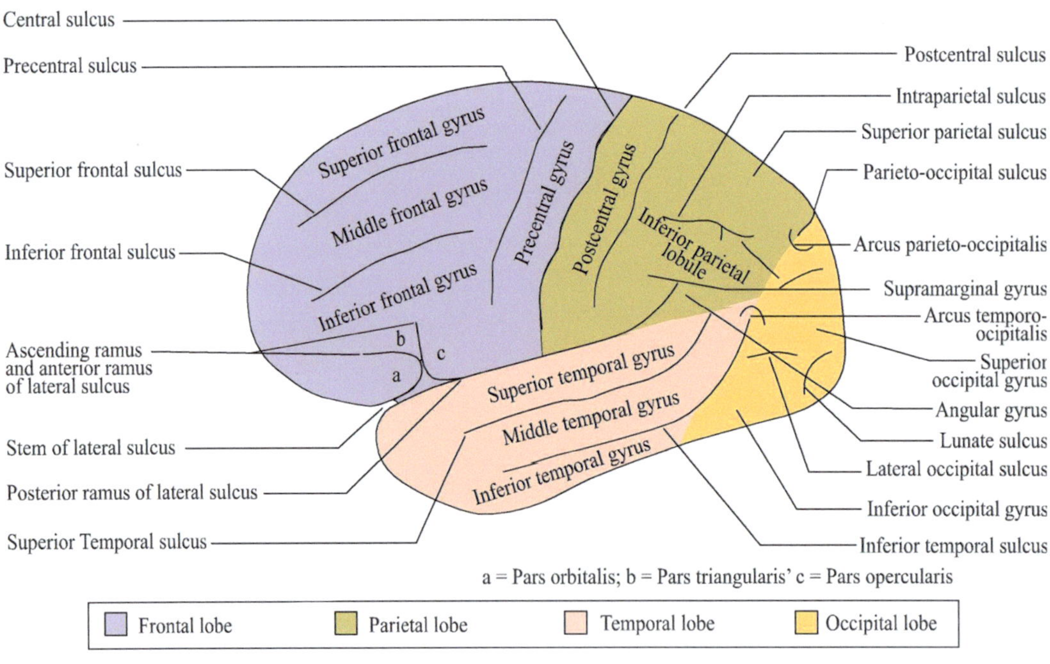

Fig 3.8 Cortex: superolateral surface

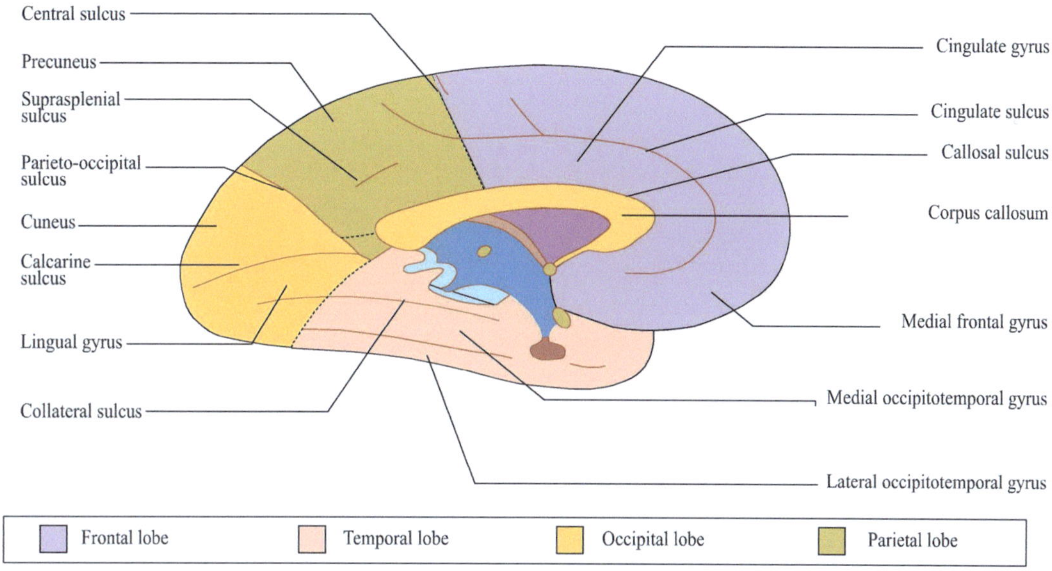

Fig 3.9 Cortex: mesial surface

Fig 3.10 Cortex: Inferior Surface

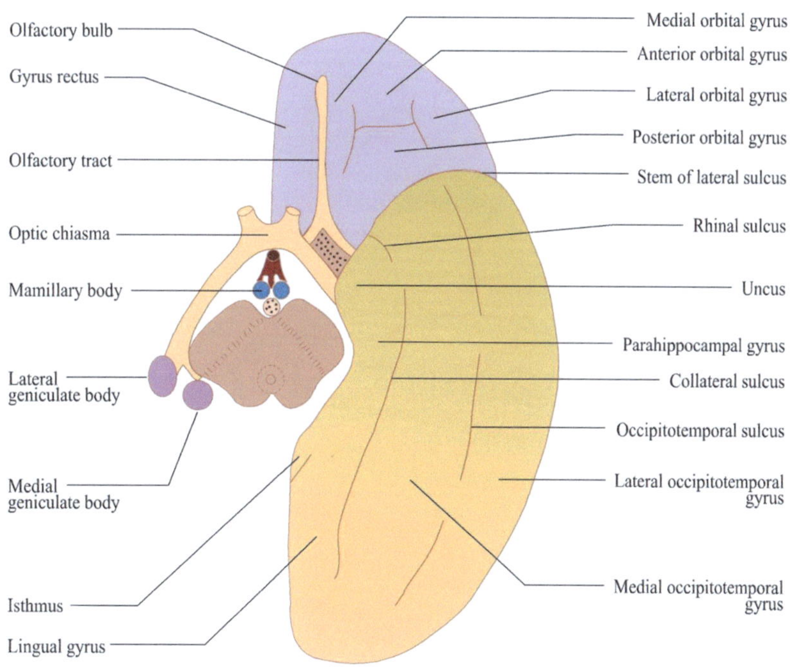

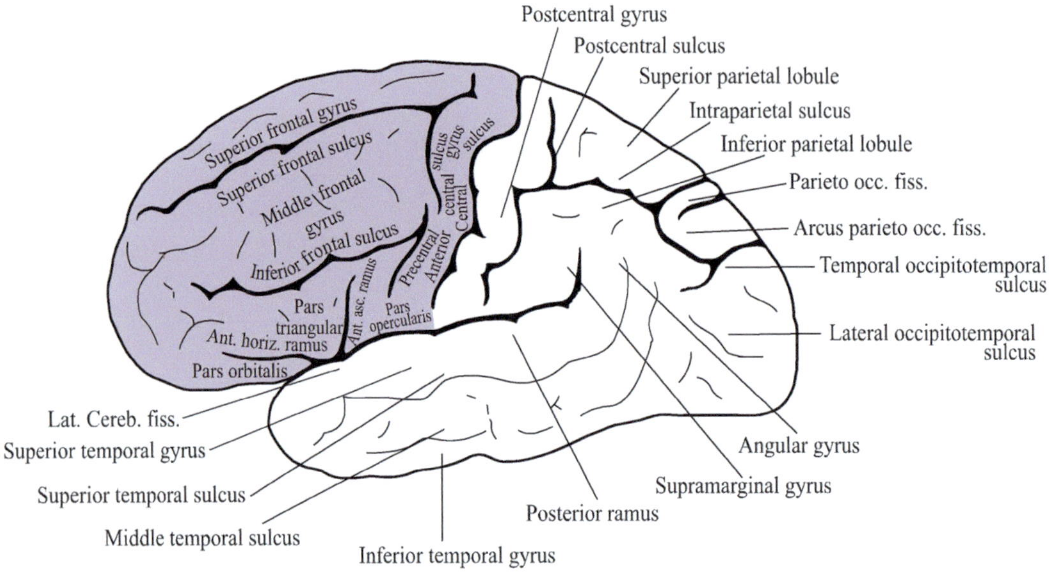

Fig. 3.11 Frontal lobe: superolateral surface

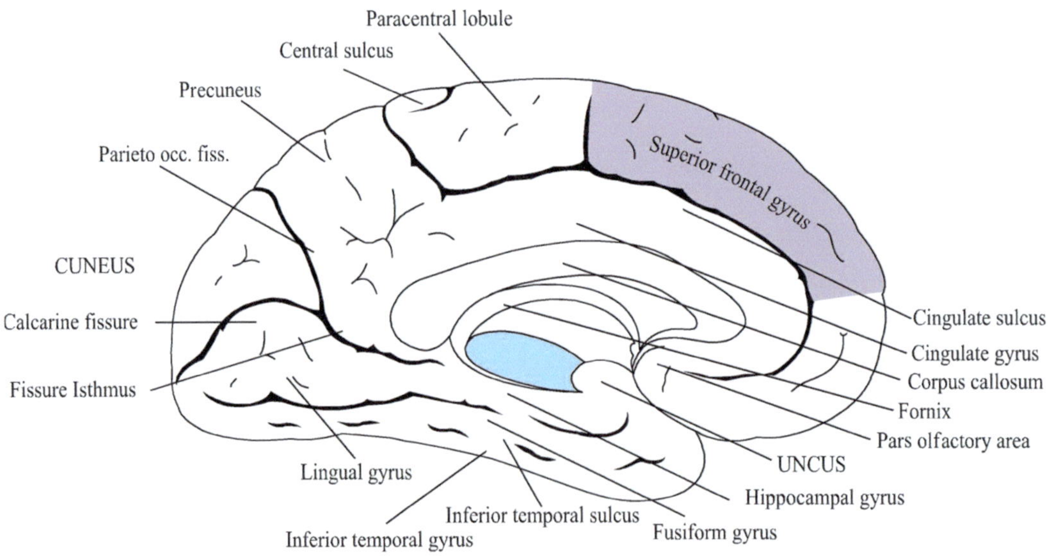

Fig. 3.12 Frontal lobe: mesial surface

3.4.3 Supplementary Motor Area (Area 6)

1. Important in planning motor movements sequentially and coordinating movements between both hands.
2. Lesion results in:
   (a) Alien hand syndrome (apraxia)
   (b) Mild hemiparesis with severe spasticity
   (c) Emergence of released reflexes

3.4.3.1 Released Reflexes

- These are primitive reflexes that are seen normally in normal babies and then disappear as the CNS matures. Frontal lobe inhibits these reflexes. These reflexes maybe normal in young babies and the elderly (when they are present bilaterally). These released reflexes are abnormal and indicate a pathology if they are elicitable unilaterally.

Grasp

Patient's hand is stroked distally across the palm on the lateral aspect of palm by the examiner's fingers. A forced grasp movement or adduction of the thumb, even when told to relax indicates a lesion of the contralateral frontal lobe area 6.

Sucking (Pout, Spout, Rooting)

Sucking—Stroke the lip of the patient with a finger resulting in sucking movements.

Snout reflex—Place the examiner's index finger on the closed lip of the patient and tap the examiner's finger with a percussion hammer or tap the patient's lip directly with the examiner's index finger resulting in pouting of lips. Indicates damage to contralateral corticobulbar fibers or lesion of the contralateral frontal lobe area 6.

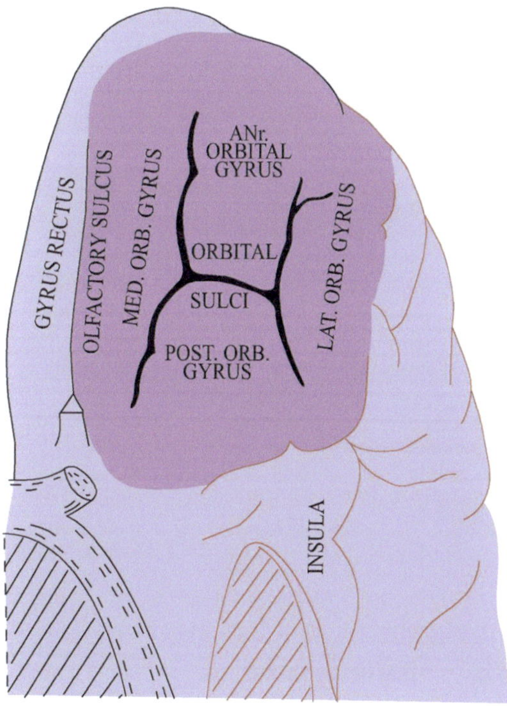

Fig. 3.13 Frontal lobe inferior surface

Palmo-Mentalis

Palm (especially thenar eminence) of the patient is gently stroked by the examiner's finger resulting in ipsilateral puckering of the skin of the chin.

Glabellar Tap

Examiner repeatedly taps the glabellar area, i.e., the center of the forehead just superior to the nose resulting in involuntary bilateral eye closure.

In normal individuals, the eye closure fatigues after 4–5 taps. In Frontal lobe disease and Parkinson's disease, the glabellar tap continues to result in eye closure without fatigue.

3.4.4 Frontal Eye Field Area (Area 8)

Controls conjugate gaze movement of the eyes to the contralateral side.

- Lesion will cause gaze palsy or impaired saccades to the contralateral side.

3.4.5 Broca's Area (Area 44)

- Lesion of Dominant lobe causes anterior (expressive) aphasia.
- Lesions of nondominant lobe results in Dysprody (loss of melody and rhythm of speech).

3.4.6 Prefrontal Lobe

Areas anterior to areas 6 and 8 and include Brodmann area 9, 10, 11, 12, 32, 45, and 47. It forms the main projection to the dorsomedial nucleus of the thalamus and to the basal ganglia. It is further subdivided into 3 parts:

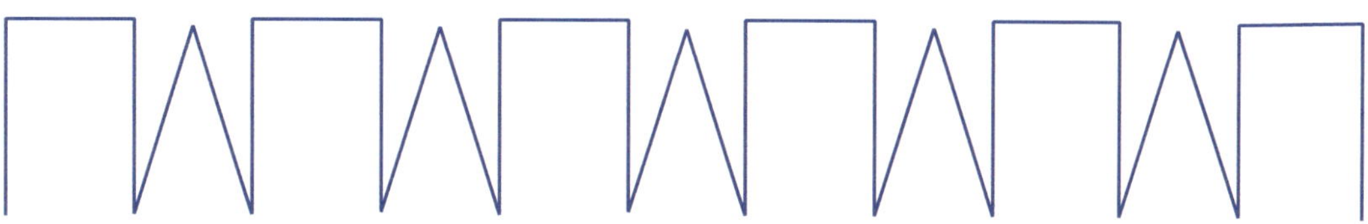

Fig 3.14 Alternating pattern

3.4.6.1 Dorsolateral Prefrontal Cortex

Lesions result in

1. Personality changes
2. Impaired executive function
   (a) List generation provides names of cities starting with letter "A" or name animals or fruits.
   (b) "Go/No Go" test—patient has to respond, e.g., by touching knee on each "go signal" and not responds to "No" signal.
   (c) Stroop test—Different names of colors are written in different colors, e.g., the word red is written in green color and the word yellow is written in blue color.

       Patient has to state *the color of the ink* and not read the word.
3. Perseveration—Difficulty in abandoning previous verbal or motor response.

3.4.6.2 Medial Prefrontal Cortex

Involvement of the paracentral lobule results in

(i) Incontinence without insight
(ii) Gait abnormality, especially apraxia of gait with short steppage narrow-based gait and marching at one point with surprisingly fairly maintained movement when making cyclical movements while lying in bed.

3.4.6.3 Orbito-Frontal Region

Lesions result in:

(i) Disinhibition syndrome
(ii) Emotional lability
(iii) Poor judgment

Function and testing

Area	Function	Test
Primary motor area (4)	• Motor function (origin of corticospinal) of contralateral limit • Somatosensory perception	• Nondense UMN hemiplegia
Supplementary motor area (6)	• Performance of smooth movement by sensorimotor integration	I. Apraxia II. More spasticity than paresis III. Released reflexes
Frontal eye field (8) Premotor area	• Saccadic contralateral • Eye movement Involved in planning and execution of movement	• Contralateral gaze palsy • Impaired saccades • Motor Luria • Ring-fist (loss of kinetic melodies) • Graphic Luria
Prefrontal area (9, 10, 11, 12, 32, 45, 47) (a) Dorsolateral Prefrontal (b) Medial prefrontal region (c) Orbitofrontal region	• Executive function • Personality	• Tests for executive function and planning • Go-no-go test • Perseveration • Incontinence • Gait abnormality • Disinhibition • Emotional lability • Poor judgment
Brocas area(44)	• Speech expression in dominant lobe	• Nonfluent aphasia • Loss of prosody in nondominant lobe
Orbital and basal area (10, 11) Anterior cingulate gyrus 24 (Mesial frontal lobe)	• Motivation and goal-directed behavior • Empathetic, civil, and socially appropriate	• Personality changes • Disinhibition • Apathy and Akinetic mutism • Incontinence without insight

3.5 Parietal Lobe

The parietal lobe is separated anteriorly from the frontal lobe by the central sulcus, laterally from the temporal lobe by the sylvian fissure, and posteriorly from the occipital lobe by the parieto-occipital sulcus (an imaginary line extending from the pre-occipital notch of the temporal lobe superiorly to the parieto-occipital sulcus). The inter-parietal sulcus runs posteriorly from the midpoint of the postcentral gyrus and separates the rest of the parietal lobe into the superior parietal lobule and the inferior parietal lobule which is further subdivided into the supramarginal gyrus and angular gyrus. Important Brodmann areas in the Parietal lobe include (Figs. 3.15 and 3.16):

- Postcentral gyrus—Area 3
- Superior parietal lobe—Area 5, 7
- Interior parietal lobe—Area 39 Angular gyrus,
- Area 40 Supramarginal gyrus

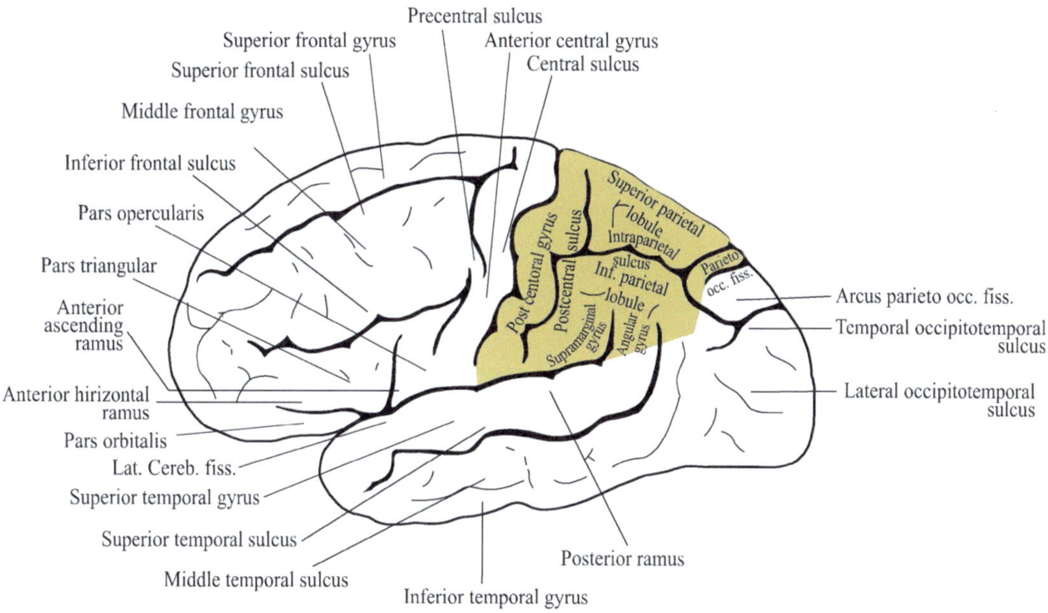

Fig 3.15 Parietal lobe: superolateral surface

Fig. 3.16 Parietal lobe: mesial surface

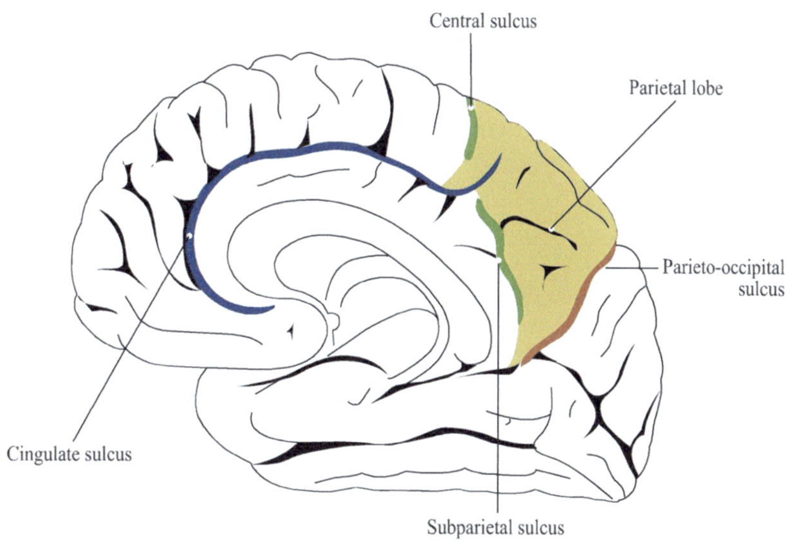

3.5.1 Functions of Parietal Lobe and Tests According to Functional Regions of the Parietal Lobe

3.5.1.1 Post-Cental Gyrus (Area 3, 1, 2)

1. Ensure intactness of basic exteroceptive and proprioceptive sensations before proceeding for cortical sensation evaluation.
2. Evaluate for 5 cortical sensations:
   (a) Astereognosis: (inability to identify objects held and felt in the patient's hand with closed eyes.)
   (b) Agraphasthesia: (inability to recognize letters written on the patients' skin at different body areas with a blunt object. Numbers like 0, 1, 3, 8, 7 where the stimulation is completed without raising the stimulus while writing the number are commonly utilized.)
   (c) Loss of two-point discrimination: The two point discriminator simultaneously touches 2 widely separated skin areas and the patient has to identify whether the stimulation is one or two different stimuli. Once the patient identifies the two point stimulation correctly, the distance between the two points is gradually reduced till the two points cannot be differentiated from one another. This distance is noted. This distance between the 2 points at which the patient can correctly observe the difference between one point or two point stimulation will be different over sensitive areas like palm and over less sensitive areas like the trunk. This distance can be compared with the contralateral side or compared with the examiners skin surface to identify whether it is normal or abnormal.
   (d) Lack of tactile localization—Patient has to identify with eyes closed, which body part has been touched.
   (e) Sensory inattention—Simultaneous stimulation on both sides and similar body regions is conducted. Sensory inattention is labelled when the patient cannot identify the simultaneous stimulation on the contralateral side though can identify when the skin on that part is stimulated without simultaneous stimulation (seen with lesions of secondary association area and more commonly in nondominant lobe).

3.5.1.2 Visual Pathway (Optic Radiation)

Results in contralateral inferior quadrantanopia or hemianopsia.

3.5.1.3 Cuneous (Medial Aspect)

Lesion results in Transcortical sensory aphasia

3.5.1.4 Superior Parietal and Inferior Parietal Lobe

Dominant Lobe Lesions

1. *Apraxia* Inability to produce skilled movement not caused by motor weakness, sensory loss, tone, posture abnormality nor poor comprehension.
   (a) *Ideomotor apraxia*
      I. Patient cannot perform the motor task and makes errors and also cannot pantomime the motor act.
   (b) *Ideational apraxia*
      I. Inability to plan multiple step motor acts with difficulty in performing sequencing of complex acts though can perform individual steps correctly.
   (c) *Limb-Kinetic apraxia*
      I. Difficulty in performing fine movement of fingers and thumb separately with appearance of clumsiness in the absence of any motor deficit. For example, picking an object between thumb and index finger or moving a coin in hand.
2. *Gertsman syndrome (Angular gyrus syndrome)* consists of:
   (a) Finger agnosia—Inability to identify various fingers
   (b) Alexia with Agraphia (difficulty in reading and writing)
   (c) Acalculia—Impaired ability to make calculations

(d) Left to right disorientation—Difficulty in identifying right from left sided limbs.

3. *Asymbolia for pain*—Abnormal reaction to painful stimulation, e.g., laughter in response to painful stimulation.

Nondominant Lobe Lesions

Constructional Apraxia

Inability to reproduce or copy 2- or 3-dimensional objects, e.g., polygonal star, 3-dimensional cube.

Dressing Apraxia

Severe difficulty in wearing clothes. Can be tested by asking the patient to wear a shirt whose one arm has been pulled inside out.

Topographic Memory Loss

Difficulty in geographic memory of the room, building, locality, state, country, and world.

Anosognosia

- Patient is unaware of the deficit.
- Maybe accompanied with or without explicit denial of the deficit and confabulation.

Hemineglect (Contralateral)

Neglect of half of the patient's body or the entire contralateral environment including that half of the body.

Hemiasomatognosia

Unilateral misperception of one's body image.

Parietal lobe lesions can also cause:

(i) Wasting of the contralateral limbs
(ii) Pseudo-cerebellar syndrome—Clumsiness simulating dysmetria
(iii) Dystonia
(iv) Pseudoathetoid (wandering) movements of contralateral limbs

	Dominant	Nondominant
Post-central gyrus (3,1 2) Primary sensory cortex	Contralateral sensory loss • Astereognosis • Agraphasthesia • Loss of two point discrimination • Lack of tactile localization	Contralateral sensory loss • Agraphasthesia Loss of two point discrimination
Secondary association Sensory area	Sensory inattention—Simultaneous stimulation on both sides, similar regions cannot be identified on contralateral side	Contralateral sensory inattention
Visual pathway (optic radiation)	Contralateral inferior quadrantanopia	Contralateral interior quadrantanopia
Cuneus (medial aspect)	Transcortical sensory aphasia	
Superior Parietal and inferior parietal lobe	1. Apraxia (a) Ideomotor apraxia Patient cannot perform the motor task and makes errors (b) *Ideational apraxia* Inability to plan multiple-step motor act with difficulty in performing sequencing of complex acts (c) *Limb-Kinetic apraxia* 2. *Gertsman syndrome (Angular gyrus)* (a) Finger agnosia (b) Alexia and Agraphia (difficulty in reading and writing) (c) Acalculia (d) Left to right disorientation	(i) *Constructional apraxia* Inability to reproduce or copy 2 or 3-dimensional objects (ii) *Dressing apraxia* Severe difficulty in wearing clothes (iii) *Topographic memory loss* Difficulty in geographic memory of room, building, locality, state, country, and world (iv) *Anosognosia* Unawareness of deficit With or without explicit denial and confabulation (v) *Hemineglect (contralateral)* Neglect of half of the body or entire contralateral environment (vi) *Hemisomatognosia* Unilateral misperception of one's body image
	• Asymbolia for pain–abnormal reaction to painful stimulation, e.g., laughter	

3.6 Temporal Lobe

Situated in the middle cranial fossa, it is situated anterior to the occipital lobe, posterior to the frontal lobe, and inferior to the sylvian fissure. The temporal lobe is subdivided into superior, middle, and inferior temporal gyri, lateral occipito-temporal, lingual, fusiform, parahippocampal, and hippocampal gyri (Figs. 3.17 and 3.18).

Auditory fibers travel from the medial geniculate body to the auditory cortex (Areas 41 and 42). Hearing is bilaterally represented with contralateral dominance and hence unilateral temporal lobe lesions do not cause hearing loss.

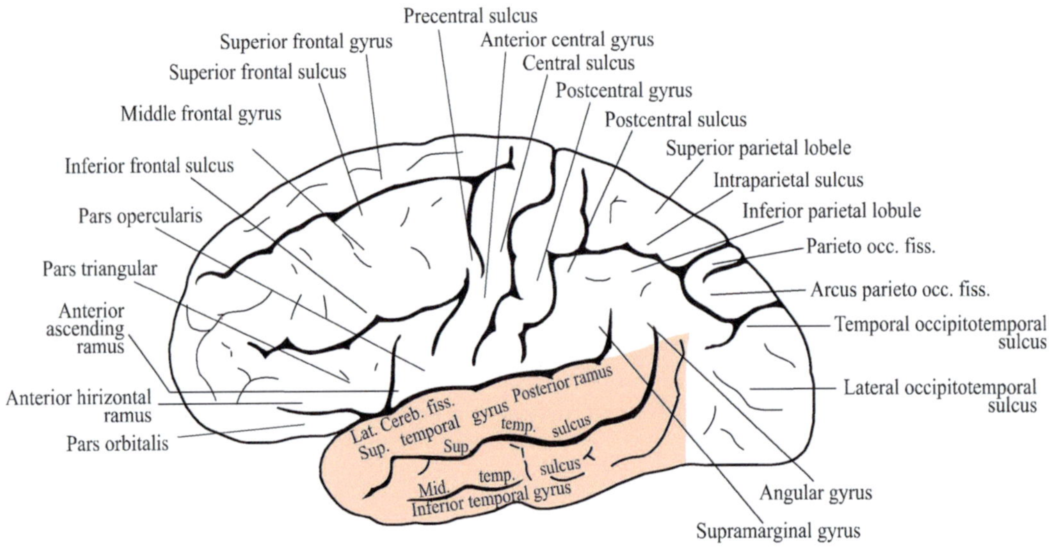

Fig. 3.17 Temporal lobe: superolateral surface

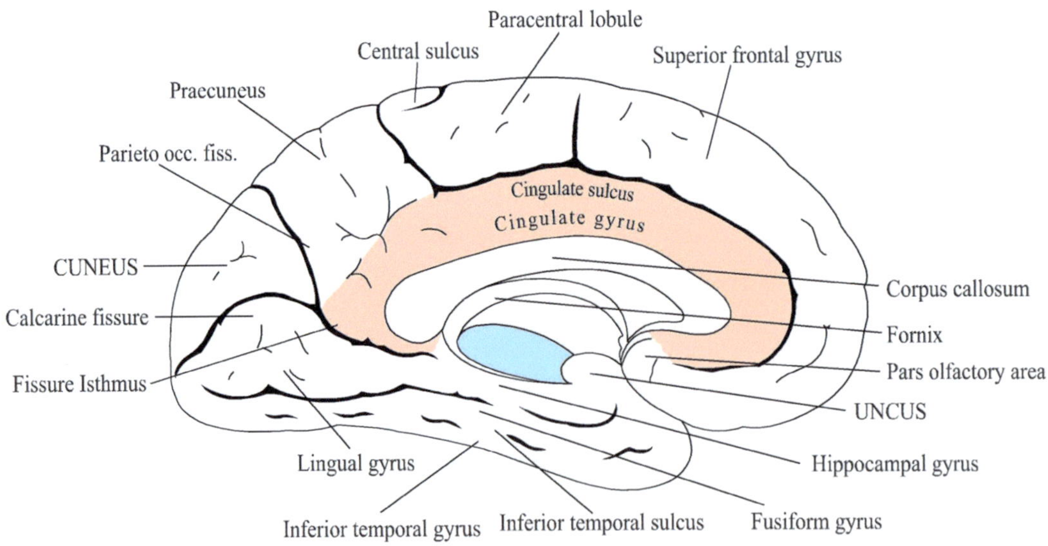

Fig. 3.18 Temporal lobe mesial aspect

3.6.1 Functions and Tests According to Functional Regions of the Temporal Lobe

1. *Primary Auditory cortex (Areas 41 and 42)*
   (a) Unilateral temporal lobe lesion does not result in hearing loss due to bilateral representation of hearing but can result in difficulty in sound localization and bilateral dulling of hearing acuity.
   (b) Bilateral temporal lobe lesions of the auditory area may lead to cortical hearing loss with or without awareness of the deficit.
   (c) Caused by dominant or bilateral temporal lobe lesions.
   (d) Auditory Agnosia—Impaired capacity to recognize known sound, e.g., bell, phone, clap even though the patient can hear the sound. It results from dominant or bilateral temporal lobe lesions.
   (e) Pure word deafness—Cannot understand spoken words though has intact reading and writing ability. It is caused by dominant or bilateral temporal lobe lesions.
   (f) Conduction aphasia—Caused by lesions of primary auditory cortex 41, 42, or supramarginal gyrus (area 40). These patients have intact fluency and comprehension but severely impaired repetition.
2. *Wernicke's Area (Area 22 posterior 2/3 of superior temporal gyrus)*
   (a) Lesions of dominant Wernicke's area will result in posterior aphasia characterized with fluent spontaneous speech with impaired comprehension.
   (b) Transcortical sensory aphasia results from lesions of posterior middle temporal gyrus (area 37) or angular gyrus (area 39). These patients have impaired comprehension but can repeat sentences (echolalia) though without understanding the content.
3. *Optic radiation*—Results in Contralateral superior hemianopsia or quadrantanopia.
4. *Infero-mesial aspect (amygdala, hippocampus)*

   Amnesia that is greater for verbal information in dominant temporal lobe lesions and greater for visuospatial information in non-dominant lobe lesions.
5. *Non-localizing features*
   (a) Auditory hallucinations and complex visual hallucinations are seen in patients with temporal lobe lesions.
   (b) Psychiatric manifestation, e.g., behavioral disorders, personality changes, emotional and mood changes, anxiety and paranoia maybe seen in patients with temporal lobe lesions.
6. *Amusia*—Inability to appreciate different characters of heard music. Dominant lobe dysfunction leads to difficulty in appreciating lyrics whereas nondominant lesions lead to impaired appreciation of rhythm and pitch of the music.
7. *Bitemporal lobe*—Lesions in animals can produce a syndrome called Kluver-Bucy syndrome manifesting with visual agnosia, hyper-orality, hyperphagia, and hypersexuality. Partial forms of the syndrome are seen in humans with bilateral temporal lobe lesions.

Area	Dominant	Nondominant
Infero-mesial aspect (amygdala, hippocampus)	Amnesia (greater for verbal information)	Amnesia (greater for visuospatial) memory
Posterior 2/3 superior temporal gyrus—Area 22/Wernicke's area	• Wernicke's Aphasia	• Sensory aprosody (poor perception of emotional overtones)
Primary auditory cortex (41,42) • Posterior middle temporal gyrus	• Pure word deafness • Word selection dysnomia • Transcortical aphasia sensory (can repeat a sentence without understanding or performing the command)	• Sensory amusia (inability to recognize familiar previously heard melodies, read musical notations, and inability to detect out of tune notes

Area	Dominant	Nondominant
Auditory agnosia	Dominant or bilateral temporal lobe	Cannot recognize sounds of clap, bell ringing, phone despite normal hearing
Non-localizing	• Auditory hallucinations • Complex visual hallucinations • Psychiatric symptoms	
Optic radiation	Contralateral superior quadrantanopia	
Bitemporal lesions	*Kluver-Bucy* syndrome • Hypersexuality • Oral exploration • Visual agnosia • Tameness	

3.7 Occipital Lobe

Occipital lobe is the smallest of the four lobes and rests on the tentorium cerebelli and is anteriorly separated from the parietal lobe and temporal lobe by the parieto-occipital sulcus (imaginary line extending from the preoccipital notch of the temporal lobe superiorly to the parieto-occipital sulcus). Only a small part of the dorsolateral surface is occupied by the occipital lobe which occupies a large part on the mesial aspect of the brain in between the parietal and temporal lobes. The Calcarine fissure divides the mesial occipital lobe surface into the cuneous above and the lingual gyrus below (Figs. 3.19 and 3.20).

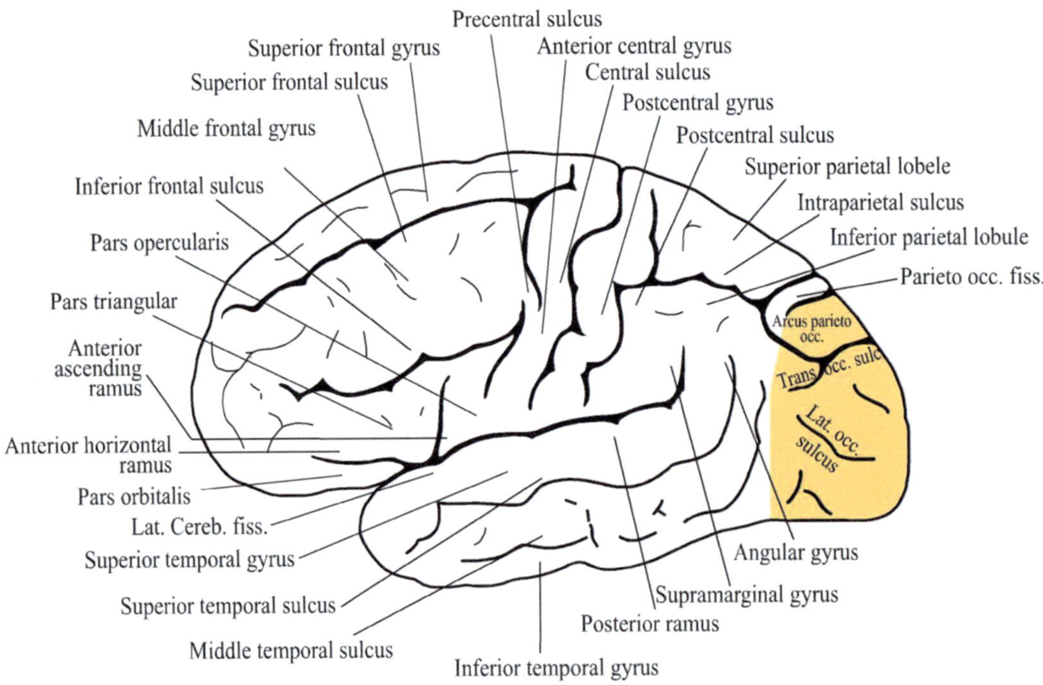

Fig. 3.19 Occipital lobe superolateral surface

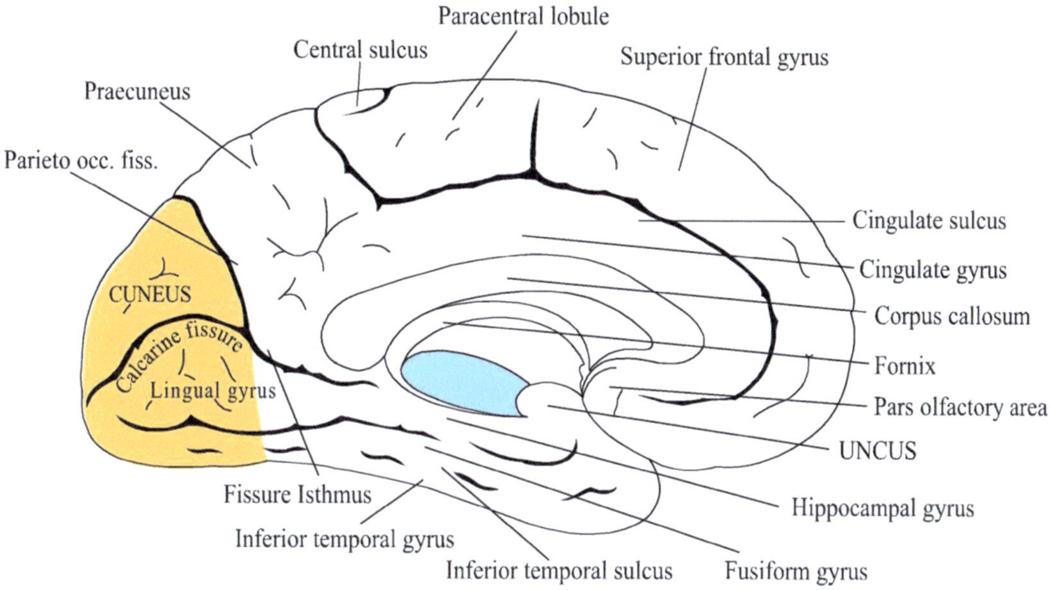

Fig. 3.20 Occipital lobe mesial surface

3.7.1 Functions and Tests According to Functional Regions of Occipital Lobe

1. *Primary visual cortex area 17* (around calcarine sulcus. Also called as the striate cortex). It receives the geniculocalcarine projection and is responsible for primary visual impressions including color, size, form, motion, and illumination.
   (a) Lesion of area 17 results in a congruous, contralateral, macular sparing, hemianopsia with preserved optokinetic nystagmus.
   (b) Color blindness—(central achromatopsia)—cannot visualize colors.
2. *Parastriate (area 18) and peristriate (area 19)* are the visual association areas and are important for recognition and identification of objects and is the seat for visual memory.
   (a) Lesions result in impaired visual memory, impaired visual localization, distorted visual images, especially distance and shape and size as well as difficulty in ocular fixation.
   (b) Simultagnosia—Inability to see a picture in its entirety and can only focus on one object in the picture at one time. Caused by lesions of dominant or bilateral area 19 lesions.
   (c) Prosopagnosia—Inability to recognize familiar faces, e.g., family or important leaders, though can recognize them by voice. Caused by lesions of nondominant or bilateral occipito-temporal lesions.
   (d) Color agnosia—Patient is not color blind as in lesions of area 17, i.e., patient can see the color and match it but cannot identify the color.

It occurs in lesions of the visual association areas.

3. *Non-localizing symptoms*
   (a) Visual hallucinations
   (b) Pallinopsia: Persistence of image even after the stimulus is removed.
   (c) Ipsilateral impaired scanning: Impaired ability to efficiently and actively looking for information relative to the environment.

4. *Bilateral occipital lobe syndromes*
   (a) *Anton's Syndrome*
      I. Bilateral hemianopsia with or without macular sparing(Cortical blindness).
      II. Pupillary light reflex is preserved.
      III. Other cortical defects, e.g., color agnosia, prosopagnosia, and simultagnosia.
      IV. Anosognosia (lack of awareness of blindness) with or without denial.
   (b) *Balint-Holmes syndrome*
      I. Optic ataxia—Normal visual acuity and fields but inability to reach for objects with visual help.
      II. Optic apraxia—Inability to voluntarily fixate and control gaze.

Occipital lobe—areas and clinical effect

Area	Dominant	Nondominant
Lateral surface	Alexia with agraphia	• Visual hallucinations • Visual field defect
Mesial surface	• Visual agnosia • Alexia without agraphia	• Visual hallucinations • Visual field defects • Contralateral homonymous hemianopsia or quadrantanopia with macular sparing • Ipsilateral impaired scanning (efficiently and actively looking for information relative to environment) • Pallinopsia (persistence of image after stimulus is removed) • Visual aesthesia
Bilateral occipital lobe lesions	*Anton syndrome* Denial of blindness with confabulation (predominantly involvement of nondominant occipital lobe and visual association areas as well as primary visual area *Balint syndrome* Optic ataxia and optic apraxia	

Cranial Nerve Examination

4

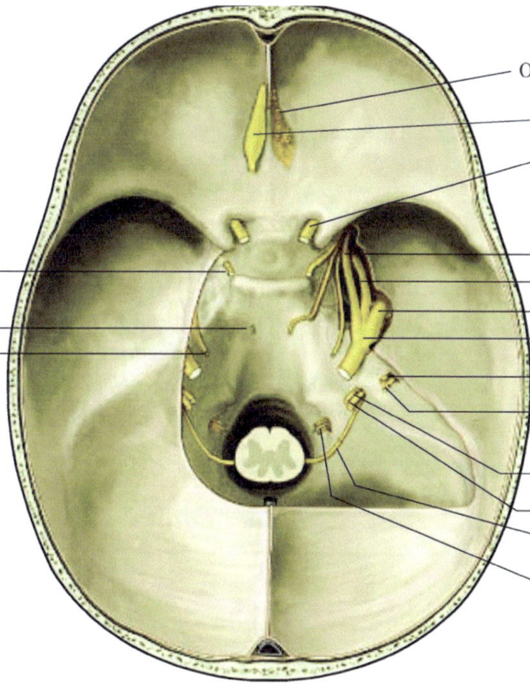

Fig. 4.1 Cranial nerves

4.1 Olfactory Nerve: 1st Cranial Nerve (Figs. 4.1)

4.1.1 Neuroanatomy (Figs. 4.2 and 4.3)

It is the shortest Cranial nerve carrying sensation of smell from the nasal mucosa to the olfactory bulb.

- First-order neurons

  16–20 million olfactory cells lie in the olfactory mucosa of the nasal mucosa and the peripheral processes of the first-order neurons carry sensation from the olfactory epithelium. The central processes of the olfactory neurons form about 20 branches on either side, which penetrate the cribriform plate and synapse with the second-order axons in the olfactory

V. Suri, *Clinical Neurological Examination and Localization*,
https://doi.org/10.1007/978-981-16-1228-2_4

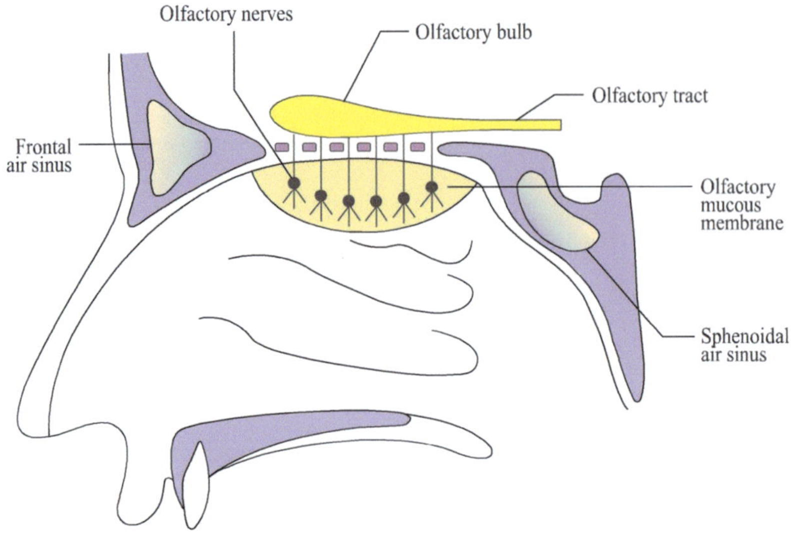

Fig. 4.2 Olfactory nerve

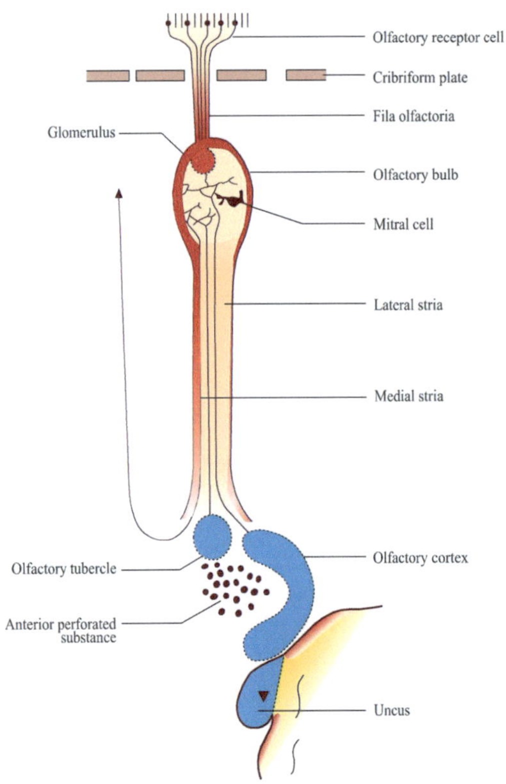

Fig. 4.3 Olfactory pathway

bulb. These *20 branches (central part of the first-order axons) crossing the cribriform plate* constitute the *olfactory nerve.*

- Second-order neurons

  Olfactory bulb gives off fibers that form the olfactory tract that reaches the primary olfactory cortex, which is constituted by the anterior perforated substance and adjacent gray matter areas.
- Fibers form the primary olfactory areas (anterior perforated substance) travel to the secondary olfactory area (entorhinal area) located in the uncus and anterior part of the Parahippocampal gyrus of the temporal lobe. Olfaction is perceived in both the primary and the secondary olfactory areas.

4.1.2 Clinical Testing

1. Exclude nasal block by asking the patient to sniff on a metal tongue depressor and ensure bilateral haze on the metal tongue depressor.
2. Small bottles (of similar shape and color) containing various smelling substances, e.g., coffee, chocolate, peppermint, and vanilla are used. Avoid irritating odors, e.g., ammonia, since it may be perceived as pain through the trigeminal nerve and be misconceived as perceiving odors. The patient is advised to take two good but not overexuberant sniffs through one nostril while closing the other nostril by external pressure. The patient is asked
   (a) Whether he/she can smell anything.
   (b) Whether he/she can identify the odor.

   The same odor is then evaluated on the other nostril and the patient is asked whether he/she can smell anything, whether he/she can identify the odor and whether he/she felt the same intensity of the smell in both the nostrils.

(a) The test is then repeated with 1 or 2 other odors after allowing an interval time to disperse the previous odor.

4.1.3 Clinical Interpretation

1. *Anosmia*—Inability to detect odor or loss of smell. It is important to identify whether the patient can perceive the odor even though he/she may not be able to identify the odor. Perceiving the odor suggests continuity of the olfactory pathway and correct identification of the odor suggests intact cortical function.

   Causes:
   (a) Local acute or chronic inflammatory nasal disease
   (b) Heavy smokers
   (c) Parkinson's disease
   (d) Past or recent head injury with olfactory nerve trauma
   (e) Basifrontal tumors, e.g., olfactory groove meningioma
   (f) Viral respiratory infections, e.g., COVID-19 viral infection
2. *Parosmia*

   Can detect the odor but all odors are distorted and appreciated as an unpleasant sensation.

   Causes:
   (a) Depression
   (b) Recovering head trauma
3. *Hyposmia*

   Patient can perceive the odor but needs stronger stimulation to perceive it compared to other individuals or compared to the contralateral nostril. Most patients with anosmia or hyposmia may complain of loss of taste rather than loss of smell since olfaction contributes a significant proportion to the flavor of food.
4. *Olfactory agnosia*
   (a) The patient is able to perceive the odor but cannot identify the odor.
   (b) Indicates intact olfactory nerve with lesion of the primary or secondary olfactory cortex.

4.2 Optic Nerve: 2nd Cranial Nerve

4.2.1 Neuroanatomy (Fig. 4.4)

- The optic nerve extends from the retina to the optic chiasm and is approximately 5 cm in length.
  - *Intraocular part*—(1 mm) at the optic disc where fibers move to retro-orbital region.
  - *Intra-orbital part*—(approximately 25 mm) from posterior aspect of the eyeball to the optic canal and is surrounded by the three meningeal layers.
  - *Intracanalicular part*—(4–10 mm) within the optic canal of the sphenoid bone.
  - *Intracranial part*—(approximately 10 mm) travels from optic canal superior to the diaphragm sella and cavernous sinus to join the contralateral nerve to form the optic chiasm.
- Macula—is the central point of fixation and comprises only of cones and hence is the site of greatest visual acuity and color perception. It is a shallow depression in the retina lying temporal to the disc (Fig. 4.5).
- Optic Disc (papilla)—is the head of the optic nerve visible through the ophthalmoscope.

4.2.2 Functions

- Transmits visual impulses from the retina to the lateral geniculate body of thalamus (visual afferent fibers).
- Pupillary afferent fibers regulating the pupillary light reflex.

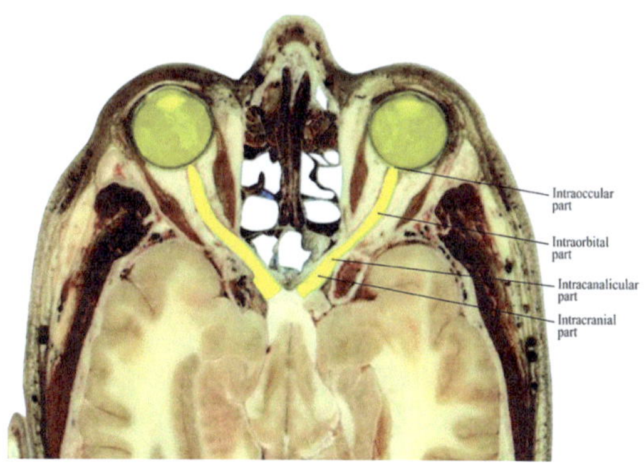

Fig. 4.4 Optic nerve

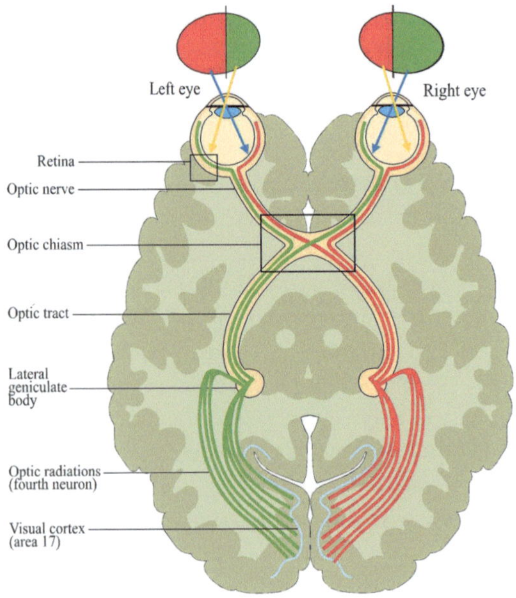

Fig. 4.5 Visual pathway

4.2.3 Clinical Testing

1. Visual acuity
2. Color vision and contrast sensitivity
3. Visual field
4. Pupillary reaction
5. Fundus

4.2.3.1 Visual Acuity

Visual acuity is impaired in optic nerve lesions

- Visual acuity is most reliably tested at 20 ft (6 m) using a standard chart, e.g., Snellen chart where the patient sits 6 m away from the chart or by a mirror at 3 m between the patient and the chart. Electronic computer screens may also be utilized.
- If the patient cannot read even the largest letter on the chart then counting fingers at 1 m or identifying hand movement at 1 m or perception of light and projection of rays is utilized.
- Near vision is recorded by reading near vision charts at a distance of 33 cm.

4.2.3.2 Color Vision

- Acquired color perception impairment, especially for red color can be affected in optic nerve disease even prior to loss of visual acuity. Patients can be evaluated by *Ishihara charts* or by showing a red bright target to one eye at a time. In the affected eye, the red color appears less bright and washed out.
- Impaired *contrast sensitivity* wherein the patient cannot differentiate between different contrasting shades of the same color may be an early sign of optic nerve disease.

4.2.3.3 Visual Field testing

Fibers from the temporal field of vision (nasal retinal fibers) cross the optic nerve and decussate to the contralateral side in the optic chiasm and travel along the contralateral optic tract and optic radiation to the contralateral occipital cortex. Fibers from the nasal field of vision (temporal retinal fibers) travel laterally in the optic nerve and in the ipsilateral optic tract and optic radiation to the ipsilateral occipital cortex.

Some fibers from the optic tract pass via the superior colliculus to the mid-brain to mediate the pupillary light reflex through the Edinger Westphal nuclei.

Hemianopsia

Impaired vision in one half of each eye with the loss not crossing the vertical meridian.

1. Homonymous hemianopsia—field loss in corresponding halves of each eye.

   Heteronymous hemianopsia—field loss in non-corresponding areas, e.g., binasal or bitemporal (in sellar lesions).
2. Homonymous hemianopsia may be similar shaped in both eyes or differently shaped (Fig. 4.6).
   (a) Congruous—similar shape of field defect in both eyes. More posterior, i.e., closer to the occipital lobe more congruous the defect.
   (b) Incongruous—different shape of field defect in both eyes. More anterior the lesion more incongruous the defect.
   (c) Macular sparing Homonymous hemianopsia—indicates lesion of occipital lobe lesion involving area 17.

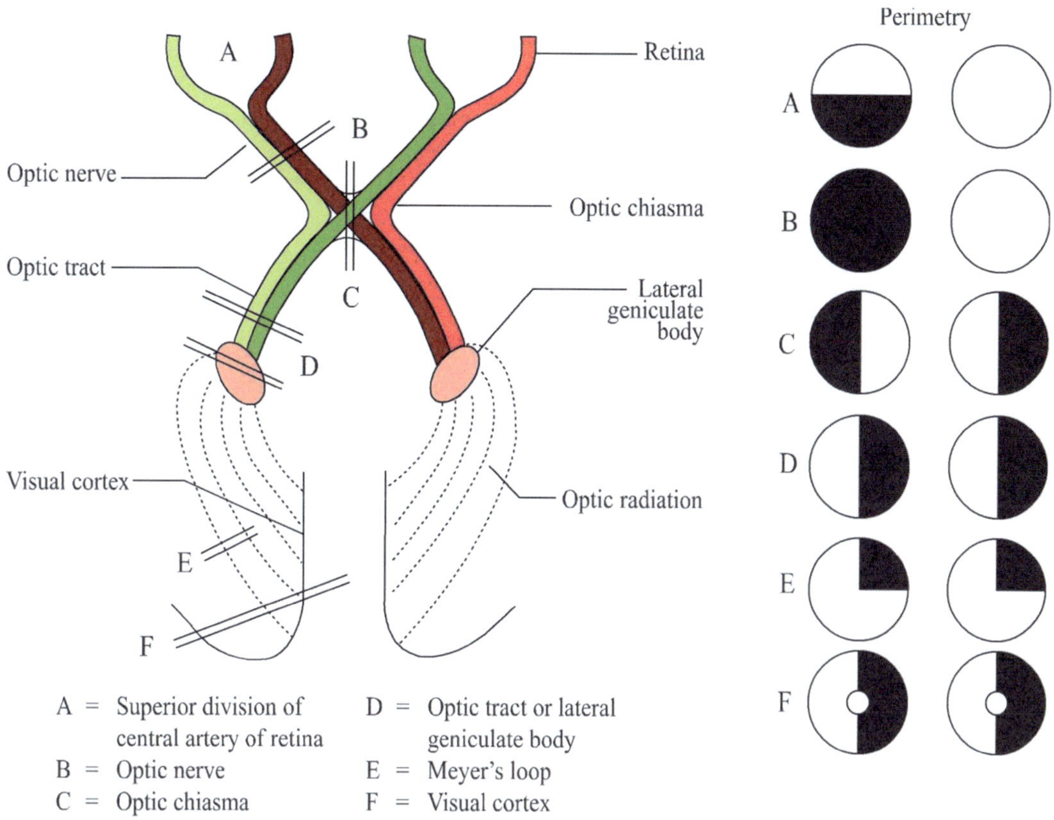

Fig. 4.6 Field defect according to site of lesion

Altitudinal defect is when the field defect involves the upper or lower half of the field without crossing the horizontal meridian. Commonly seen in retinal vascular disorders, e.g., central retinal artery occlusion, retinal artery branch, or occlusion or anterior ischemic optic neuropathy.

Optic nerve lesion causes unilateral vision loss.

Optic chiasmal lesion causes bitemporal or unilateral temporal field defect.

Retro-chiasmal lesions cause homonymous (i.e., equivalent part of temporal field in one eye and nasal field of contralateral eye) hemianopsia. Homonymous hemianopsia can be non-congruent (bilateral field defect is unmatched) in *optic tract* lesion or congruent (matched bilateral field defect) in *occipital cortex* lesions where macular sparing is an additional finding.

Optic radiation lesion in temporal lobe can result in a superior homonymous quadrantanopic and parietal lobe radiation lesion can cause inferior homonymous hemianopsia.

Field charting can be conducted by:

- *Goldman perimetry*
- *Automated Humphrey fields*
- *Bedside confrontation testing*—patient and examiner sit at the same level 1 m apart and the patient is instructed to look at the examiner's eyes. Patient's field is compared to the examiner's field by moving or wriggling the examiner's index finger in all peripheral and central fields one eye at a time (other eye closed). Simultaneous stimulation in both eyes to assess for visual inattention should be conducted at the end of the examination.

4.2.3.4 Pupil

Assess size of pupil (normal 2–4 mm), shape of pupil (round, oval, or irregular) and position (central or eccentric) and assessment of the response of pupil to light and accommodation is of extreme importance in localizing visual pathway lesions.

Pupillary constriction is a parasympathetic function. The afferent pathway for the light reflex travels along the visual pathway from the retina and crosses from the optic tract via the superior colliculus to the mid-brain Edinger Westphal parasympathetic nucleus. Efferent fibers travel from the Edinger Westphal nucleus into the oculomotor nerve to the ciliary ganglion from where second-order neurons innervate the pupillary sphincter. These pupillary fibers are peripheral in the oculomotor nerve and hence extrinsic compression of the 3rd nerve, e.g., by a posterior communicating aneurysm will affect these fibers resulting in 3rd nerve lesion with dilated pupil whereas microvascular ischemic lesion of the 3rd nerve, e.g., in diabetes will cause 3rd nerve palsy with normal pupil.

Pupillary dilation is a sympathetic function. The first-order neurons originate from the hypothalamus and travel along the brainstem and cervical cord to the ciliospinal center in the lower cervical and upper dorsal cord from where second-order neurons travel via T1 root and sympathetic chain to the superior cervical ganglion. Third-order neurons travel from the superior cervical ganglion along the internal carotid artery up to the cavernous sinus region and then to the orbit to supply the pupillary fibers and the Mullers muscle. Lesion anywhere in the sympathetic pathway from the hypothalamus, brainstem, cervical or upper dorsal cord, or the superior cervical ganglion or the third-order neurons can result in Horner's (miosis, ptosis, enophthalmos, anhidrosis, and loss of ciliospinal reflex).

Clinical Testing

- Check pupil size in normal illumination (12% of persons may have some mild anisocoria though with normal reaction to light and accommodation).
- Check pupillary reaction to light using a bright torch, by direct response (in eye where light stimulation is performed) and using the examiner's left hand as a barrier on the patient's nose to shield the other eye from the light source. This is followed by testing for the consensual response (contralateral eye stimulation with light and evaluating pupil response in ipsilateral eye). Constriction of the pupil should be brisk and sustained.
- *Afferent pupillary defect* suggestive of optic nerve dysfunction will result in absent ipsilateral direct reflex with brisk and sustained consensual response in the ipsilateral eye on contralateral stimulation.
- *Accommodation reflex* is evaluated by asking the patient to look distantly and then focus on the examiner's finger advanced to 20 cm from the patient's eyes. Observe for constriction of the pupil as the eyes converge onto the examiner's finger close to the patient's eye.

4.2.3.5 Fundus Examination (Fig. 4.7)

Fundus evaluation for various disorders affecting the disc or retina, e.g., papilledema, optic atrophy, optic neuritis, retinal degeneration, or retinopathy can be conducted by

- Direct ophthalmoscopy
- Slit lamp evaluation

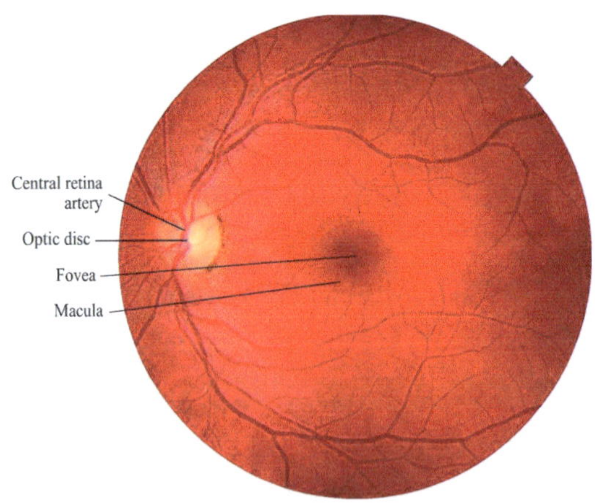

Fig. 4.7 Normal fundus

Direct ophthalmoscopy allows visualization of the optic disc and retina and its circulation by a 15× magnified image.

Pupil is preferably dilated with 1% tropicamide and patient is requested to fixate on a distant object after dimming the room lights and setting the lens to zero (except to correct the examiners refractory disorder). Use examiner's right eye to examine patient's right eye and examiner's left eye to examine the patient's left eye.

Evaluate:

1. *Disc*—First examine the disc which is usually, immediately visible if the patient is looking at a distance. If the disc is not visible follow the vessels to their convergence where the disc can be visualized.
   (a) Color—pink or pale (atrophy) or hyperemic (neuritis, papilledema).
   (b) Margins—distinct or indistinct (papilledema)—keep in mind that nasal blurring may be a normal finding in normal individuals and hence blurring of the temporal side with absence of venous pulsations should be considered as an early sign of papilledema.
   (c) Venous pulsations—abolished in papilledema.
   (d) Physiological cup—obliterated or normal.
2. *Vessels*
   (a) Arteries are lighter and narrower than veins and often have a central reflecting "silver wire line."
   (b) Arteries may have thickening of walls with obliteration of veins at points of crossing (A V nipping) and variable widening and narrowing of lumen in hypertensive patients.
   (c) Venous engorgement and loss of pulsations may be an early sign of increased intracranial pressure or central vein thrombosis (Figs. 4.8 and 4.9).
3. *Retina*
   (a) Hemorrhage—streaks or flame-shaped or large ecchymosis.
   (b) Exudates—Cotton wool, fluffy appearing exudates are focal microinfarcts and may be seen in papilledema, renal failure, vasculitis, retinal embolism, and severe anemia.
   (c) Tubercles—usually seen as rounded lesions with yellow center and ill-defined pink edges are marginally elevated and about half the size of the disc (Figs. 4.10 and 4.11).

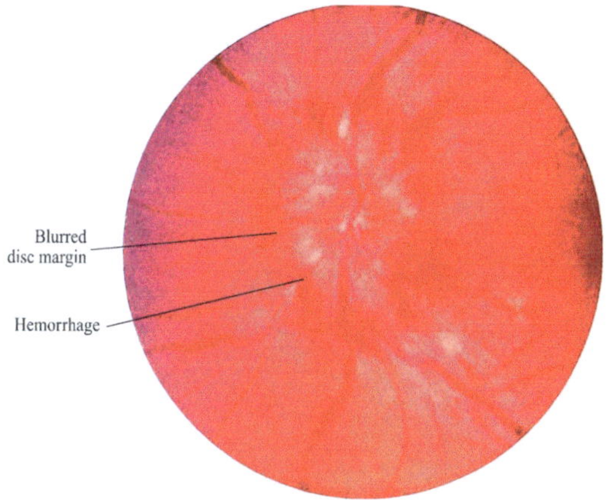

Fig. 4.8 Papilloedema

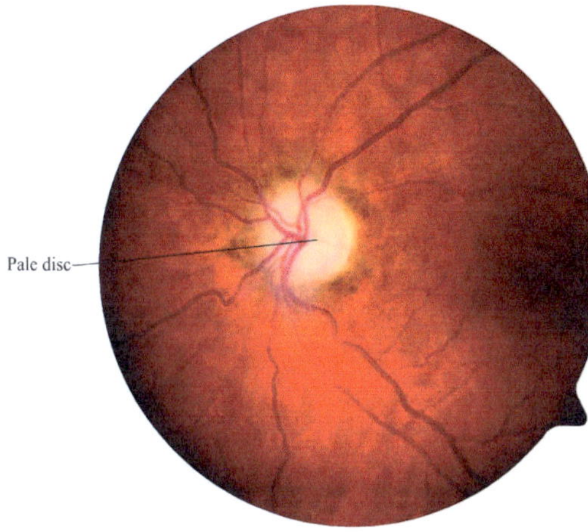

Fig. 4.9 Optic atrophy

4.2.4 Fluorescein Angiography

Fluorescein angiography is a diagnostic procedure in which 10% fluorescein is injected intravenously and photographs are taken to study the circulation of the retina and choroid.

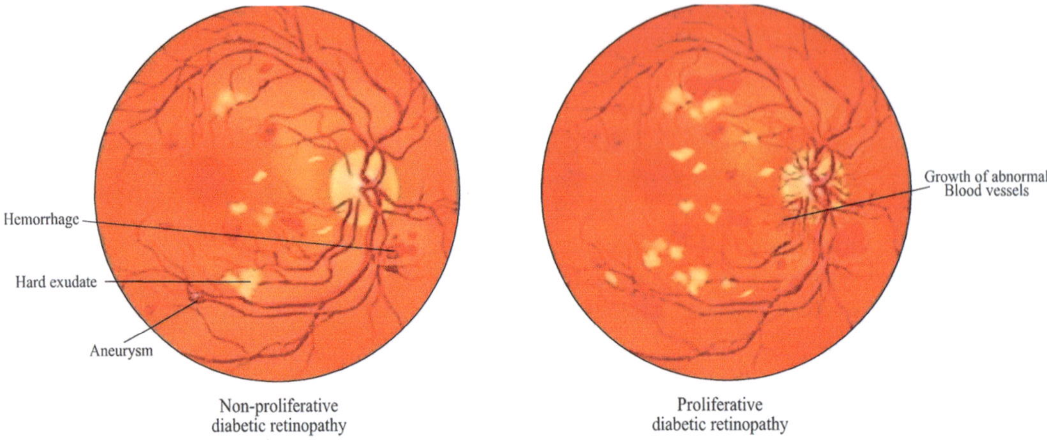

Fig. 4.10 Diabetic retinopathy

Fig. 4.11 Hypertensive retinopathy

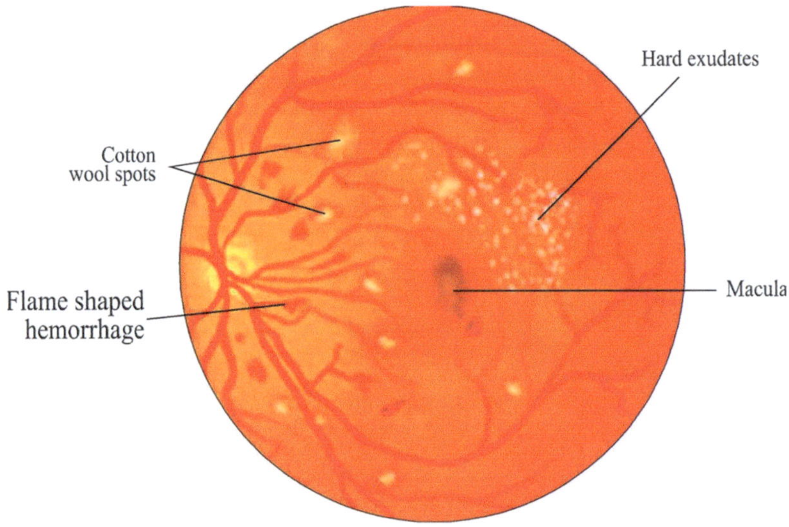

Fluorescein does not escape from normal arterioles but may extravasate from the arterioles in patients with papilledema (but not in pseudo—papilledema) and in central venous occlusion.

4.2.5 Optical Coherence Tomography (OCT)

OCT is a noninvasive diagnostic procedure used for imaging the retina and utilizes light waves to take cross section images of the retina. It provides high-resolution cross section images of the retina, retinal nerve fiber layer, and the optic nerve head.

It is used for imaging of the macula, optic nerve, and choroid and is helpful in patients with age-related macular degeneration, central serous chorioretinopathy, diabetic retinopathy, intraocular hemorrhage, papilledema, and inherited retinal disease.

4.3 Oculomotor (3rd), Trochlear (4th), and Abducens (6th) Cranial Nerves

4.3.1 Neuroanatomy

Ocular movements are controlled from the frontal eye field area with output to the paramedian pontine reticular formation and medial longitudinal fasciculus in the brain stem which controls the 3rd, 4th, and 6th nuclei, and then pass through the individual cranial nerves and through the neuromuscular junction to the orbital muscles.

Four cortical areas that are connected to each other generate the saccadic (rapid) movement to the contralateral side. These areas include the Frontal eye field area (area 8), supplementary eye field area which is part of the supplementary motor area, the dorsolateral prefrontal area, and the parietal posterior eye field area. Fibers from these centers descend to the Pontine paramedian reticular formation (PPRF which predominantly activates the 6th nerve nucleus) and the Medial longitudinal fasciculus (MLF which predominantly activates the 3rd and 4th nerve nuclei). The PPRF and MLF coordinate horizontal conjugate movements by coordinating the action of the ocular nuclei in the brainstem. The vertical movements in the brainstem are controlled in the midbrain by the rostral interstitial nucleus of Medial longitudinal fasciculus (riMLF). The medial part of the riMLF regulates the downgaze and the lateral part regulates upgaze. Individual nerves then travel from the individual nuclei to supply the ocular muscles through the neuromuscular junction.

Hence, lesions at any point from cortex to subcortical structures including the brainstem or individual cranial nerves, neuromuscular junction, or orbital muscles themselves can result in ocular movement disturbances.

- Lesions of the supranuclear pathways or brain stem result in disturbances of gaze (gaze palsies involving bilateral eyes).
- Whereas intranuclear lesions of nuclei in brainstem or cranial nerves or NM junction or ocular muscle itself cause individual or multiple ocular muscle weakness.

Some of the important terminologies of ocular movements need to be understood:

Abduction—horizontal lateral movement of eyeball.

Adduction—horizontal medial movement of eyeball.

Elevation—vertical upward movement of eyeball.

Depression—vertical downward movement.

Intorsion—rotation with upper part of eye moving medially.

Extorsion—rotation with upper part of eye moving laterally.

Skew deviation—vertical misalignment of eyes due to brainstem pathology.

Saccades—rapid eye movement from one point to another.

Pursuit—slow eye movement for maintaining eye fixation on a moving object.

Vestibulo-ocular reflex movements—eye movements in opposite direction to head movement in order to compensate for head movement in order to maintain fixation.

Convergence—adduction of both eyes to maintain fixation on an object close to the eyes.

Ptosis—normally the eyelid covers only one-fifth of the upper cornea. Covering more than one-fifth is labeled as ptosis and when the lid does not cover the cornea with a visible sleeve of sclera between the lid and the cornea it is labeled as lid retraction.

- Ptosis should be differentiated from ptylosis (heavy lid causing pseudoptosis). Ptosis may occur from weakness to the levator palpabrae superioris (3rd nerve) or a sympathetic lesion resulting in weakness of the Muller's muscle where the lid can be raised voluntarily without overactivity of the frontal muscle.

Enophthalmos (abnormal inward positioning of globe in the socket) is commonly seen in Horner's syndrome or due to congenitally maldeveloped eye.

Exophthalmos—abnormal outward projection of the globe in the socket.Enophthalmos and Exophthalmos are examined by looking down at both eyes from above the vertex of the head by standing behind the patient and assessing the appearance of the globe into visibility from behind the forehead brow of the patient. Precise measurement of exophthalmos or enophthalmos would require an ophthalmological consultation and measurement by an exophthalmometer.

- Unilateral exophthalmos may occur due to retro-orbital neoplasm or granulomas and bilateral exophthalmos is seen commonly in thyrotoxicosis.

4.3.2 Supranuclear Ocular Movements

Ocular movements can be subdivided into four subtypes, viz. Saccades, Pursuit, vestibulo-ocular, and convergence.

Eye movement	Characteristics	Site of control	Abnormalities
Saccades	Fast movement	Frontal lobe	Slow or broken saccades
Pursuit	Slow following object movement	Middle temporal and medial superior temporal	
Vestibular ocular	Compensatory eye movement in response to head movement	Cerebellar and vestibular nuclei	
Conver-gence	Adduction to fix on object close to the eye	Midbrain	Failure of convergence

4.3.3 Saccades

1. Conjugate rapid eye movements. Latency of saccades is 200–250 ms and velocity varies from 30 to 700 °/s.
2. Saccades are generated in the Frontal eye field area (area 8) and superior colliculus from where fibers travel through the internal capsule, reticular formation adjacent to the cerebral peduncles and end in the Paramedian pontine reticular formation (PPRF) and Rostral interstitial nucleus of medial longitudinal fasciculus (riMLF) and the fibers decussate at the level of the midbrain. Saccadic control from the cerebral cortex to the midbrain is hence contraversive, i.e., left frontal eye field area controls saccadic movement to the right.
3. Clinical testing is performed by asking the patient to rapidly look to left, right, up and down or alternatively to look at the examiner's nose, and rapidly turn eyes to the examiner's finger held at 30° in different directions.

   Observe for

   (a) Latency of the saccade
   (b) Accuracy of the saccade, e.g., hypometric saccade when it falls short of the target or hypermetric saccade when the movement overshoots the target.

4.3.4 Pursuit

- Slow, continuous, conjugate eye movements, which occur when vision is tracked on a slow moving object.
- Latency of pursuit is 120 ms and pursuit is accurate up to a velocity of 30°.
- Pursuit is generated in the medial temporal and medial superior temporal lobe.
- Clinical testing is performed by asking the patient to follow a pencil held in the examiner's hand, which is slowly moved in all directions and the patient tracks it. Saccadic pursuit is an abnormality when the smooth pursuit is replaced by multiple overlapping saccades.

4.3.5 Convergence

- Dysconjugate eye movements producing convergence of both eyes.
- Latency is 160 ms with a velocity of 20°/ms.
- Controlled by the Striate and peristriate cortex and parietal lobe with fibers reaching the pretectal area in the tegmentum of the midbrain.

4.3.6 Vestibular Eye Movements

- These movements stabilize gaze during head movement.
- Vestibular movements have a latency of 160 ms and a velocity of 300 ms.
- Sensory organs for vestibular eye movements include the semicircular canals, utricle, and saccule.

4.3.7 Nystagmus

- Nystagmus is defined as rhythmic, involuntary, oscillations of one or both eyes.
- Nystagmus should be differentiated from nystagmoid movements also called as physiological nystagmus, which occurs at extreme of gaze. Nystagmus should hence be evaluated with a deviation of eyes of less than 30°.
- As a rule the nystagmus is named after the fast phase of the nystagmus which is analogous to the saccade and is followed by a slow phase which is analogous to the pursuit movement.
- Nystagmus is best observed by focusing on the blood vessels of the sclera since it provides the most accurate observation of the type of movement of the eye, especially when the movement is rotatory.
- Record the position of the eyes when nystagmus occurs and the deviation, which produces the greatest amplitude of nystagmus.

4.3.7.1 Pendular Nystagmus

- Movement is slow in both directions with equal amplitude and is seen commonly in patients with poor vision or congenital nystagmus.
- Pendular nystagmus is central in origin from brainstem or cerebellum.

4.3.7.2 Jerk Nystagmus

- Slow phase in one direction with fast corrective phase in opposite direction and by convention the nystagmus direction is labeled by the direction of the fast phase.
- Jerk nystagmus may be horizontal, vertical, or rotatory. Jerk nystagmus may be localized to be originating from central or peripheral origin.

	Central nystagmus	Peripheral nystagmus
Sustained/ fatiguable	Sustained	Fatiguable
Associated vertigo	Absent or mild	Severe
Reduced by fixation	Absent	Present

1. *Rotatory nystagmus*
   (a) Usually of central origin.
   (b) Involves torsional or rotatory movement with slow corrective phase.
2. *Vertical nystagmus*—the movements are in vertical plane even with horizontal eye movements.
   (a) *Upbeat nystagmus*
      (i) Upbeating fast phase in primary gaze
      (ii) Indicates brainstem or cerebellar vermis lesion
   (b) *Downbeat nystagmus*
      (i) Downbeating fast phase in primary gaze.
      (ii) Indicates cervico-medullary junction lesion, e.g., Arnold chiari malformation, syringobulbia, craniovertebral abnormalities.
3. *Horizontal nystagmus*
   (a) Horizontal nystagmus is labelled when the to and fro ocular movements are in the horizontal direction.
   (b) They may originate from peripheral (labyrinthine) origin or from central origin (brainstem nuclei or connections).

4.3.8 Non-nystagmus Ocular Oscillatory Movements

1. *Ocular bobbing*
   (a) Rapid downward jerky movement of both eyes with slow drift back in primary position.
   (b) Caused by lesions of pons.
2. *Ocular flutter*
   (a) Rapid horizontal small amplitude, horizontal back-to–back saccades causing a quivering horizontal movement spontaneously or after fixation.
   (b) Caused by lesions of cerebellum or cerebellar connections or brainstem.
3. *Opsoclonus*
   (a) Continuous, involuntary, random, and chaotic saccades in multiple directions and also called dancing eyes.
   (b) Caused by lesions of cerebellum or cerebellar connections or brainstem.

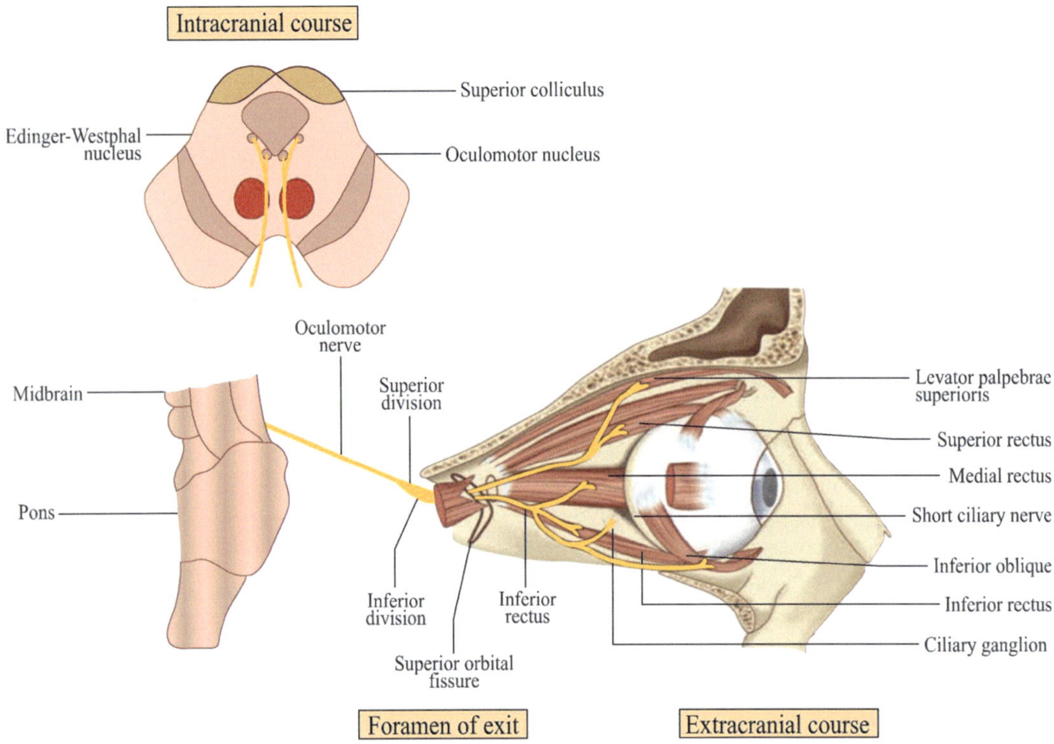

Fig. 4.12 Actions of extraocular muscles with eye in primary position

4. *Ocular dysmetria*
   (a) Overshoot or undershoot of gaze during changes in fixation.
   (b) Seen in cerebellar disorders.
5. *Ocular Dipping*
   (a) Slow downward movement is followed by a rapid return to the primary position and is also called inverse bobbing.
   (b) Seen in various encephalopathies (Fig. 4.12).

4.4 Ooculomotor or 3rd Cranial Nerve

It provides

1. Motor supply (somatic afferent) from oculomotor nucleus in midbrain to extraocular muscles—levator palpebrae superioris, superior rectus, inferior rectus, medial rectus, and inferior oblique.
2. Parasympathetic (general visceral efferent) from Edinger Westphal nucleus in midbrain to sphincter pupillae and ciliary muscles of the eye for pupillary constriction.
3. Sympathetic—no direct function but some sympathetic fibers run with the oculomotor nerve to innervate the superior tarsal muscle (Muller's muscle) for raising the eyelid.

The oculomotor nerve originates from the Oculomotor and Edinger Westphal nucleus located in the midbrain ventral to the cerebral aqueduct. The nerve emerges on the anterior aspect of the midbrain passing inferior to the posterior cerebral artery and superior to the superior cerebellar artery. The nerve then pierces the dura mater and enters the lateral aspect of the cavernous sinus within the cavernous sinus region where it receives the sympathetic branches from the internal carotid plexus, which do not enter the 3rd nerve but travel along. The nerve leaves the cranial cavity to reach the orbit via the superior orbital fissure and at this junction it divides into:

- Superior branch—supplies superior rectus and levator palpabrae superioris and carries the sympathetic supply.
- Inferior branch—innervates the inferior rectus, medial rectus, inferior oblique, and parasympathetic supply to ciliary ganglion, which innervates the sphincter pupillae and ciliary muscles (Figs. 4.13, 4.14 and 4.15).

4.5 Trochlear Nerve 4th Cranial Nerve

The Trochlear nerve is a:

- Pure motor nerve innervating a single muscle (superior oblique).
- Has the longest intracranial course though is the smallest cranial nerve (by a number of axons).
- Has a dorsal exit from the brainstem.
- It arises from the trochlear nucleus of the midbrain emerges from the posterior aspect of the midbrain and then runs anteriorly and inferiorly within the subarachnoid space before piercing the dura mater adjacent to the posterior clinoid process of the sphenoid bone.
- The nerve then moves along the lateral wall of the cavernous sinus and enters the orbit through the superior orbital fissure to supply the superior oblique muscle.
- The tendon of the superior oblique is tethered by a fibrous structure called the trochlear giving the name to the nerve. The superior oblique depresses and intorts the eyeball.
- Paralysis results in vertically separated diplopia especially in inferior gaze, e.g., reading and climbing downstairs and patients usually keeps the head tilted away from the side of paralysis (Figs. 4.16 and 4.17).

4.6 Abducens or 6th Cranial Nerve

The sixth cranial nerve like the fourth nerve has a pure somatic efferent function of supplying a single ocular muscle—the lateral rectus.

The nerve arises from the abducens nucleus in the pons and enters the subarachnoid space and pierces the dura mater to travel in the Dorrelo's canal. At the tip of the petrous temporal bone, the nerve leaves the Dorrelo's canal and enters the cavernous sinus and then enters the orbit through the superior orbital fissure where it innervates the

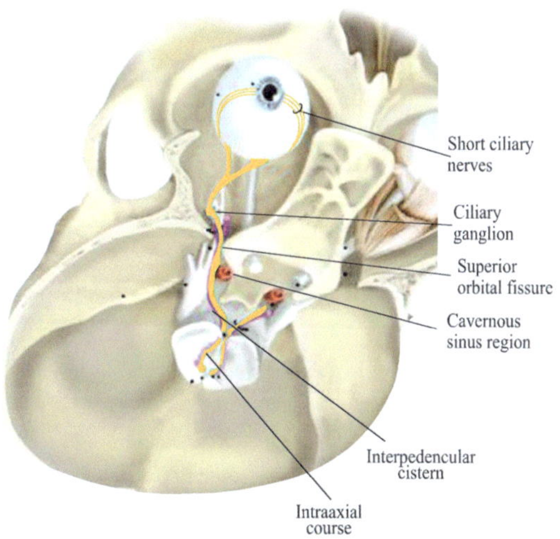

Fig. 4.13 Occulomotor nerve: origin and course

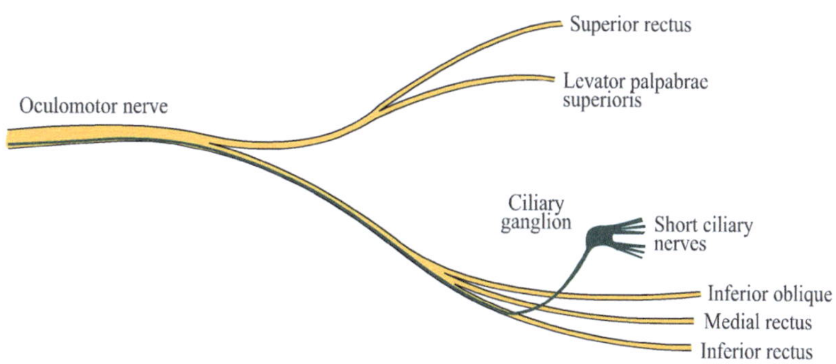

Fig. 4.14 Occulomotor nerve: course

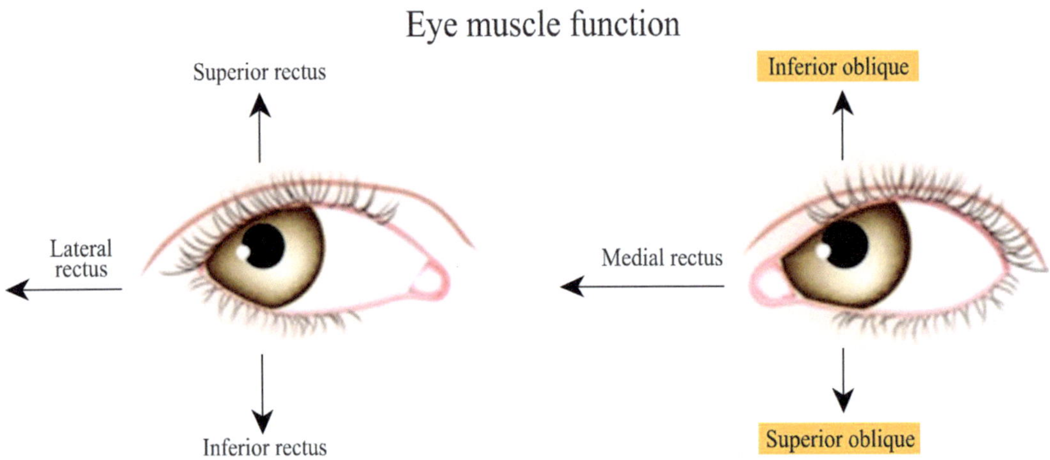

Muscle	Primary action	Secondary action
Lateral rectus	Abduction	-
Medial rectus	Adduction	-
Superior rectus	Elevation	Intorsion
Inferior rectus	Depression	Extorsion
Superior oblique	Intorsion	Depression
Inferior oblique	Extorsion	Elevation

Fig. 4.15 Occulomotor nerve: branches

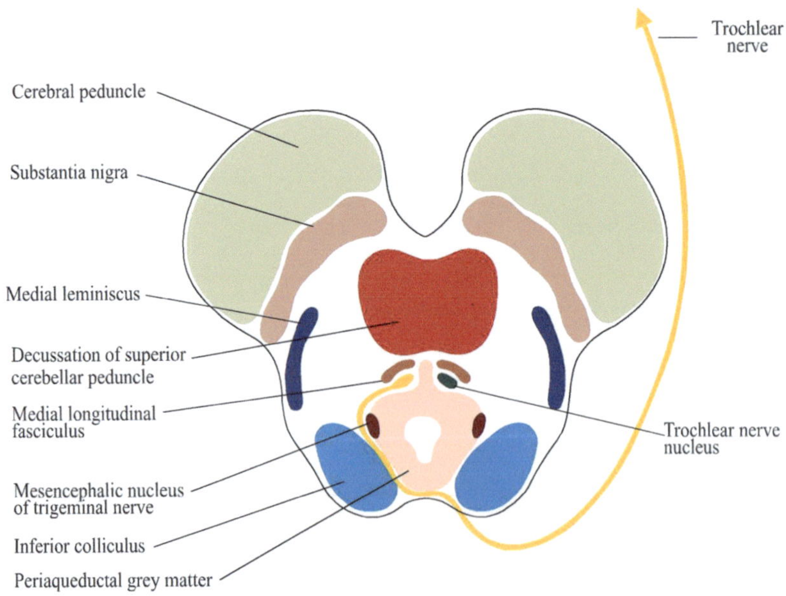

Fig. 4.16 Trochlear nerve: origin

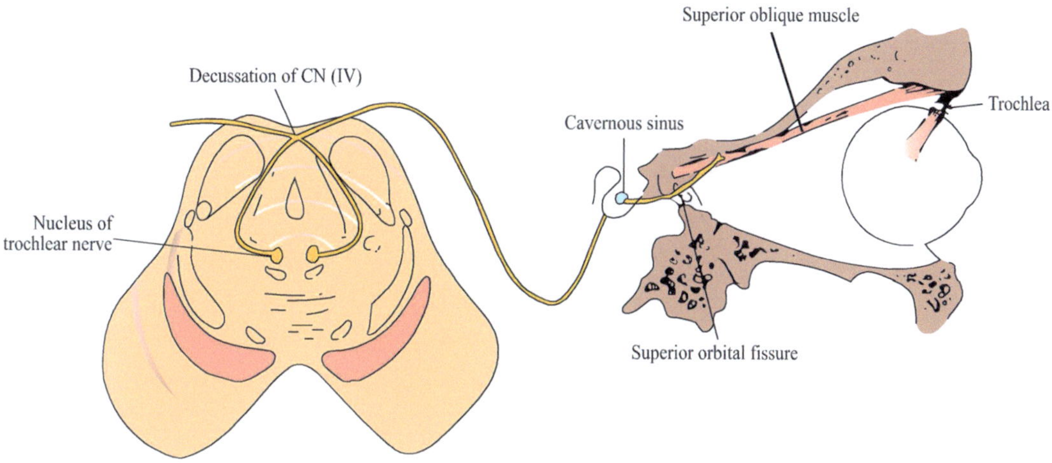

Fig. 4.17 Trochlear nerve: origin and course

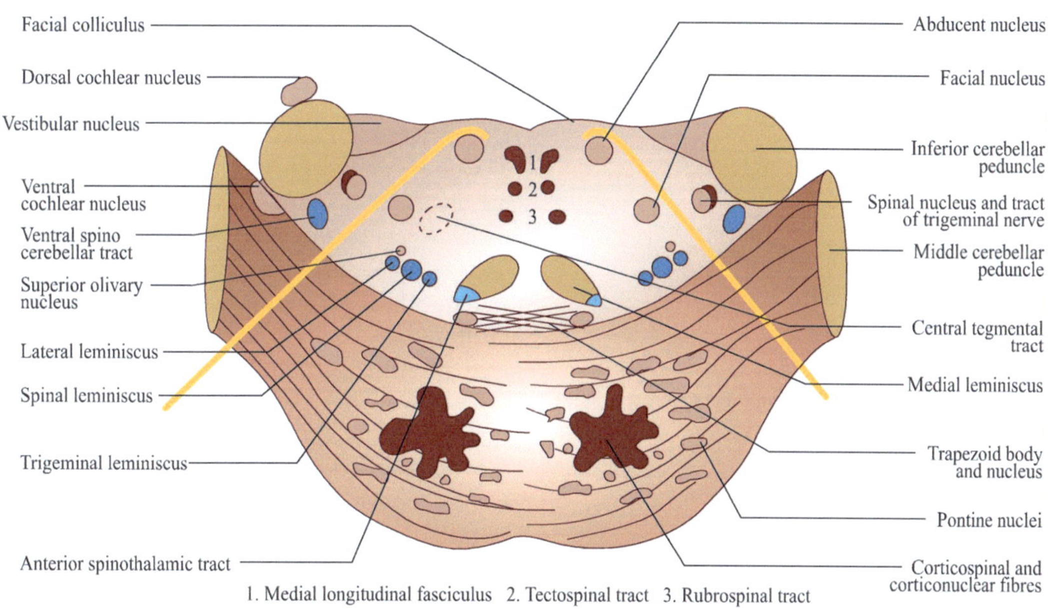

Fig. 4.18 Section through lower pons showing origin of Abducens nerve

lateral rectus muscle. The lateral rectus abducts the eyeball (Figs. 4.18, 4.19 and 4.20).

4.6.1 Clinical Evaluation

4.6.1.1 Ocular Movements

Patient is seated in front of the examiner and asked to keep the head still and follow the movement of the examiner's index finger, which is held at a distance of half a meter from the patient. Assess the primary gaze position and pursuit eye movements as the eye is moved in all directions, i.e., upward, downward, outward, inward, and in convergence.

4.6.1.2 Diplopia Testing

Patient with minimal weakness of ocular muscles may complain of diplopia and may not have any visible restriction of ocular movements. These

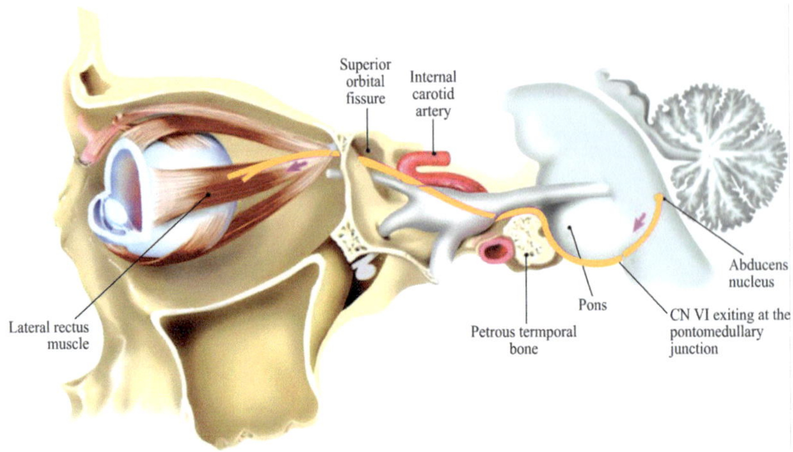

Fig. 4.19 Abducens nerve: origin and course

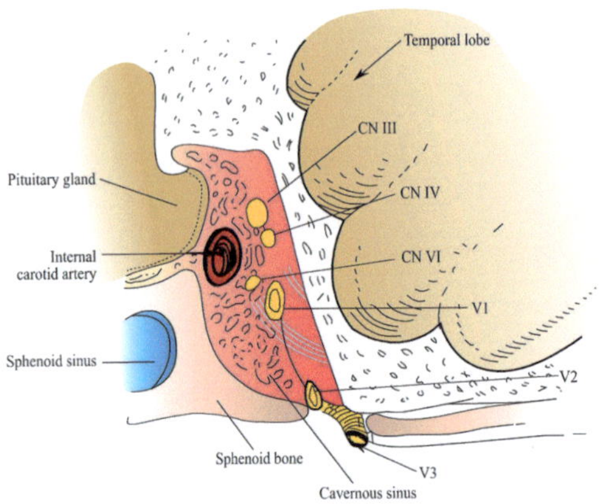

Fig. 4.20 Cranial nerves in relation to Cavernous sinus

patients will need further evaluation to determine the involved muscle/nerve.

- Assess whether diplopia is monocular (cause in one eye) or binocular.
- Determine in which direction of gaze is the diplopia maximal with maximal separation of the true and false image.
- False image is the outer image and arises from the affected eye.

Evaluate the patient sitting in front of the examiners with the head still.

- Evaluate for any corrective head tilt, e.g., tilting away from the side of the 4th nerve palsy.
- Evaluate for eye position in primary gaze and any divergence or convergence (horizontal axis).
- Skew deviation (vertical axis).

Cover Test for Latent Squint Evaluate which eye gaze produces the maximal diplopia by asking the patient to move the eye in all eight positions. Keeping the gaze in the direction of maximal diplopia, cover each eye in turn and enquire which of the two images disappear. The involved muscle is in the eye which when covered results in the disappearance of the false counter image.

4.6.1.3 Saccadic Eye Movement

- Ask the patient to quickly move eyes to the right, left, up, and down and then keep one hand in the primary position of gaze and the other hand in extreme gaze on one side and ask the patient to quickly turn eyes between both hands fixing wherever the hand is moving. In this manner can evaluate saccadic movements to right, left, up, and downward gaze.
- This test of saccadic movement can also provide evidence of a specific ocular muscle paresis.
- Next check the saccadic velocity in all directions. Slow saccades to the left would indicate a lesion in the right frontal eye field area or right internal capsule or right thalamus or

right mesencephalic reticular formation or the left PPRF.

- *Pursuit m*ovements are examined by asking the patient to follow the examiner's slowly moving finger in all directions. It also reveals any ocular paresis. It may reveal "saccadic pursuit" where the pursuit cannot keep up with the examiner's slow-moving finger and saccades overlap to keep up with the moving finger. This saccadic pursuit is commonly seen in extrapyramidal lesions, e.g., Parkinson's disease.

4.6.1.4 Evaluate Convergence

Ask the patient to look at a distant object and then at the examiner's index finger placed 50 cm from the face of the patient and then move the index finger closer to the eyes. Observe for adduction of both eyes and constriction of the pupil (accommodation reflex).

4.6.1.5 Vestibulo-Ocular Reflex (Dolls Eye Movement)

Ask the patient to fix his/her gaze at an object. Passively move the head horizontally to right and to left and vertically up and down and observe for eyeball movement in the opposite direction to the head movement. This can also be conducted in unconscious patients without fixation. Preserved dolls eye movement indicates a supranuclear pathway lesion responsible for the gaze palsy.

4.6.1.6 Evaluation of Nystagmus

- Assess for nystagmus in primary position. Concentrate on the scleral blood vessels to identify the direction of nystagmus.
- Ask the patient to move the eyes to follow the examiner's finger in all directions. Avoid evaluation in extreme gaze to avoid elicitation of physiological end point nystagmus. Preferably assess only at 30° away from the primary position in all directions.
- Assess whether nystagmus is pendular
- (symmetrical with same speed in both directions) or jerk nystagmus (slow phase and corrective fast phase). Assess whether the fast phase is in horizontal axis, vertical axis (upbeat or downbeat), or rotatory.
- Assess whether the jerk nystagmus is peripheral or central (presence or absence of vertigo, fatigability, and improvement with visual fixation).

4.6.2 Clinical Interpretation

1. *6th nerve palsy (LR6)*
   (a) Horizontally separated diplopia worsening on abduction of the eye.
   (b) Restriction of abduction of eye.
2. *4th nerve palsy (SO4)*
   (a) Vertically separated diplopia worsens on looking down.
   (b) Impaired inferior movement in adducted position and impaired intorsion.
3. *3rd nerve palsy*
   (a) Vertically separated diplopia is reported.
   (b) Ptosis, mydriasis, eyeball placed down and out with difficulty in adduction and elevation and depression of the eyeball.
   (c) Pupillary fibers are superficially placed in the 3rd nerve and hence extrinsic compression, e.g., by posterior communicating artery (PCOM) aneurysm results in mydriasis by involving the peripherally placed pupillary fibers whereas diabetic ischemic neuropathy which is non-compressive with the involvement of central fibers of the 3rd nerve due to ischemia, will have sparing of the pupil.
4. *Ophthalmoplegia*
   (a) Ophthalmoplegia refers to paralysis of one or more ocular muscles and may occur due to ocular, neurological, or endocrine causes.
      (i) Internal ophthalmoplegia—involvement limited to ciliary muscles or pupillary sphincter resulting in pupillary abnormalities with spared muscles of ocular movement.
      (ii) External ophthalmoplegia—involvement of extra-ocular muscles with sparing of pupillary sphincter and ciliary muscle.

5. *Conjugate gaze palsies*
   (a) *Supranuclear conjugate palsy*
      (i) The frontal eye field (area 8) controls contralateral conjugate eye movement and a lesion from the frontal eye field, corona radiate, internal capsule, basal ganglia, thalamus, and mesencephalic reticular formation proximal to the PPRF will result in contralateral gaze palsy.
      (ii) *Supranuclear gaze palsy*—gaze paresis originating from supranuclear lesions is accompanied with preserved vestibular-ocular reflex. Hence, intact ocular movements in the paretic gaze by moving the head with eye fixation indicates a supranuclear lesion.
   (b) *Infranuclear gaze palsy*
      (i) *Infranuclear or nuclear lesions*
      May involve the ocular nuclei or PPRF or MLF or riMLF and result in various ocular abnormalities:
      - *Conjugate gaze palsy to the ipsilateral side*. Thus, a right gaze palsy may occur from a lesion in the left frontal eye field area (supranuclear conjugate gaze palsy) or by a lesion of the right PPRF (infranuclear conjugate gaze palsy).
      - *Internuclear Ophthalmoplegia*
        Horizontal plane abnormality due to a lesion of the medial longitudinal fasciculus resulting in failure of adduction of ipsilateral eye and nystagmus in abduction position in contralateral eye.
      - *One and a half syndrome*
        Lesion of medial pons involving ipsilateral PPRF and contralateral crossing MLF.
        Gaze palsy and INO on the same side, e.g., left mesial pontine lesion will cause left gaze palsy from left PPRF and left INO from left MLF lesion leading to complete left gaze palsy and inability to adduct the left eye to the right.
6. *Skew deviation*
   (a) Vertical malalignment of both the eyes with one eye being higher or lower than the other.
   (b) Supranuclear and nuclear lesions disrupting the tracts to vertical oculomotor nucleus and the interstitial nucleus of Cajal in the brainstem and cerebellum result in skew deviation.
   (c) The lesion is usually ipsilateral to the hypotropic or lower eye.

4.7 Trigeminal or 5th Cranial Nerve

4.7.1 Neuroanatomy

The trigeminal is the largest and most complex of the 12 cranial nerves. It is a mixed motor and sensory nerve and supplies sensation to the face, mucous membranes, and motor supply to the muscles of mastication and exits the brain by a large sensory root and smaller motor root coming out of the pons at its junction with the middle cerebral peduncle.

4.7.2 Sensory Component

Sensations of pain, temperature, and touch from the face, mucous membrane of nose and cheek, tongue, and paranasal sinuses travel along the axons to the gasserian ganglion lying at the apex of the petrous temporal bone in the dural cave called the Meckel's cave.

Peripheral processes from the gasserian ganglion form three divisions:

- *Ophthalmic (V1)*—passes through the cavernous sinus and the superior orbital fissure to the orbit.

- *Maxillary (V2)*— passes through the cavernous sinus and then through the Foramen Rotundum.
- *Mandibular (V3)* which is the largest division and carries both the sensory and the motor component and exits the skull through the foramen ovale.

The central processes from the gasserian ganglion reach the sensory nucleus of the pons. Pain and temperature sensations travel to the descending spinal nucleus with tract of 5th which travels up to the upper dorsal cord.

4.7.3 Motor Component

The motor fibers arise from the motor nucleus in the pons and travel in the motor root of the trigeminal nerve bypasses the trigeminal ganglion and enters the mandibular nerve, which exits the skull through the foramen ovale and supplies the temporalis, masseter, lateral pterygoids, and four other muscles including the tensor veli palatani, tensor tympani, mylohyoid, and anterior belly of digastric (Figs. 4.21, 4.22, and 4.23).

Fig. 4.21 Section through superior pons showing origin of trigemianl nerve

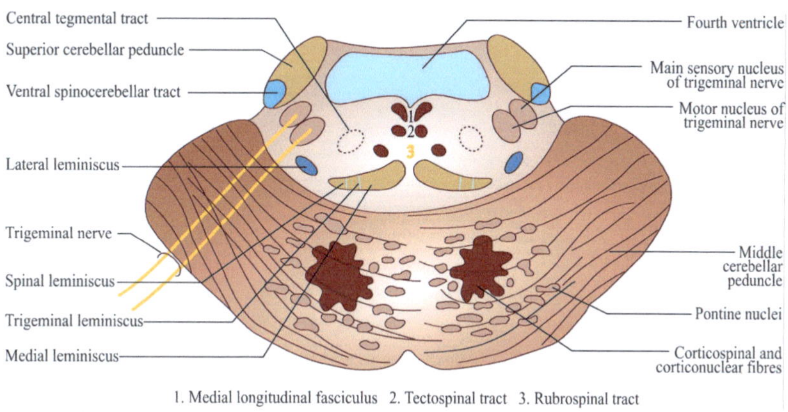

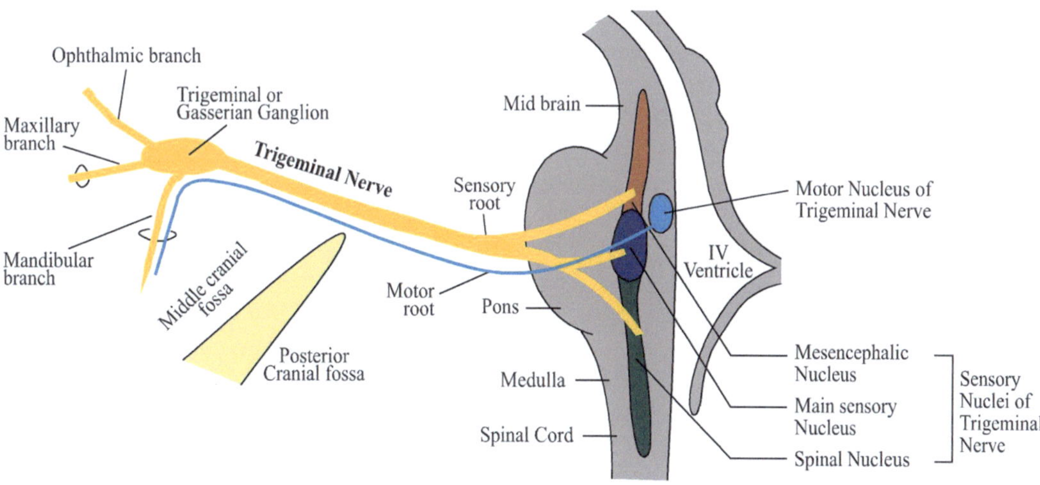

Fig. 4.22 Trigeminal nerve: origin and course

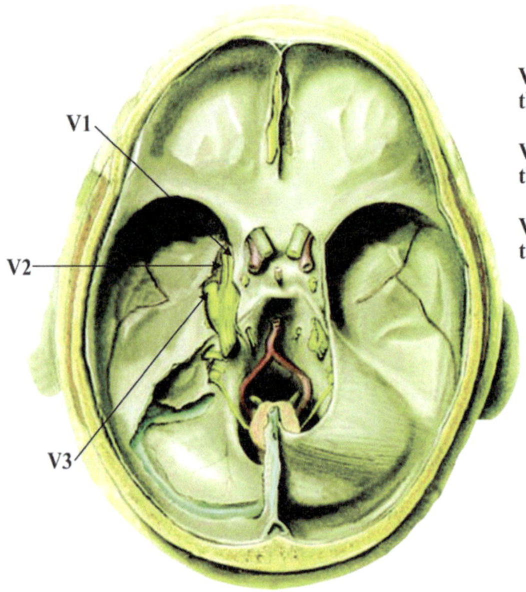

Fig. 4.23 Trigeminal nerve: branches

4.7.4 Clinical Evaluation

1. *Motor examination*
   (a) Evaluate the bulk and motor power of the temporalis and masseter muscles. Evaluate for loss of bulk in the region of the temporalis and masseter.
   (b) Feel the contraction of the temporalis and masseter muscle on asking the patient to clench the jaws.
   (c) Ask the patient to open the jaw against the examiner's hand and evaluate for deviation of the jaw toward the paralyzed side due to paralysis of the lateral pterygoid muscle (Note: Both tongue and jaw are pushed to the paralyzed side by the normal muscle).
   (d) Check for strength of the lateral pterygoid by pushing the examiner's hand with the open jaw pushing laterally.
   (e) Evaluation of other muscles including mylohyoid, anterior belly of digastric, is difficult, and maybe indicated by flaccidity of the floor of the mouth on palpation.
   (f) The palatal arch may be lower than the normal side due to weakness of the tensor veli palatini.
   (g) Difficulty in hearing and dysacusis, especially for high tones may manifest from paralysis of tensor tympani.
2. *Sensory testing*
   (a) Test for light touch with a cotton wisp and pain (pin prick) and temperature in all three divisions of the trigeminal nerve. Assess whether the sensation is felt equally in all the divisions and both sides. Also, importantly assess not only the skin of the face but also the nostrils, tongue, inner side of cheeks, and gums.
   (b) Loss of touch and pain/temperature in all divisions—lesion of gasserian ganglion or sensory root.
   (c) Loss of all modalities in one division—lesion of division in its intracranial course.
      (i) Ophthalmic division or V1—cavernous sinus and superior orbital fissure.
      (ii) Maxillary division or V2—cavernous sinus and foramen rotundum.
      (iii) Mandibular division or V3—foramen ovale.
   (d) Loss of light touch only—lesion of sensory nucleus or root in pons.
   (e) Loss of pinprick and temperature on face with intact light touch (dissociated anesthesia)—descending spinal sensory

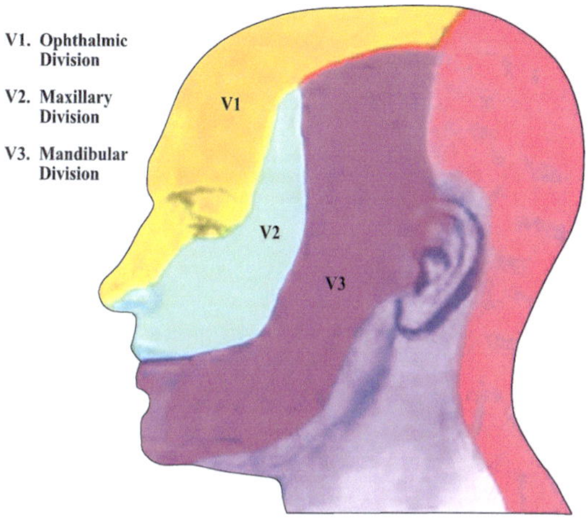

Fig. 4.24 Trigemial nerve: sensory supply on face

nucleus and tract from pons up to clinical upper dorsal cord (Fig. 4.24).

3. *Reflex testing*
   (a) *Corneal reflex*
      (i) Afferent—ophthalmic division of 5th nerve.
      Efferent—7th nerve.
      (ii) Ask the patient to look up and away so as to open the eye widely. Explain to the patient what is going to be done.
      (iii) Using the corner of a clean tissue or cotton wisp approaching from the side, touch briskly the cornea, especially the superior part of the cornea (avoid stimulating the pupil area since it would produce blinking due to elicitation of the menace reflex).
      (iv) Watch for brisk blinking bilaterally.
      (v) In 5th nerve lesion—stimulation of the paralyzed side will not elicit a blink reflex on both sides.
      (vi) In 7th nerve palsy—stimulation on the paralyzed side will elicit a blink on the contralateral non-paralyzed side with absent on ipsilateral side.
   (b) *Jaw jerk*
      (i) It is a monosynaptic muscle stretch reflex.
      (ii) Afferent—sensory portion of 5th nerve.

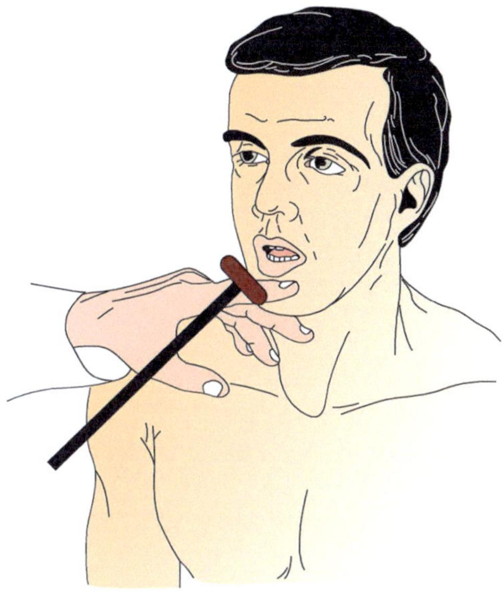

Fig. 4.25 Jaw jerk

      (iii) Efferent—motor portion of the mandibular division of 5th nerve.
      (iv) Elicited by requesting the patient to loosely sag open the jaw slightly and placing the examiner's finger below and parallel to the lower lip and tapping the examiner's finger in a downward direction with a percussion hammer.
      (v) Normal reflex—upward jerking of jaw.
      Abnormality:
      - Absent (no movement).
      - Minimal movement (normal, preserved).
      - Brisk movement (brisk jaw jerk) in lesions above the motor nucleus in pons, e.g., pseudobulbar palsy (Fig. 4.25).
   (c) *Sneezing reflex*
      (i) Afferent—ophthalmic division of 5th nerve.
      Efferent—5th, 7th, 9th, and 10th.
      (ii) Nasal mucosa is stimulated with a cotton wisp or edge of tissue. Normal response leads to a normal sneezing response.

Reflex	Afferent limb	Efferent limb
Corneal reflex	Ophthalmic division of 5th nerve	Facial nerve
Jaw jerk	Mandibular division of 5th nerve (sensory portion)	Mandibular division (motor) of 5th nerve
Sneezing reflex	Maxillary division of 5th nerve	Vagus nerve
Lacrimation reflex	Ophthalmic division of 5th nerve	Facial nerve

Site of lesion	5th related deficit	Accompanying neurological findings
Supranuclear 5th pathway		
1. Lesions of contralateral sensory cortex, corona radiata, internal capsule, or VPM thalamic nucleus	Hemifacial sensory loss	• Cortical signs of apraxia, agnosia • Hemisensory loss of sensations
2. Midbrain	Contralateral hemifacial sensory loss	• Crossed hemiplegia • 3rd, 4th cranial nerve palsy
Nuclear lesion (nucleus of 5th)		
1. Pons	Ipsilateral hemifacial sensory loss (onion peel distribution may be seen)	• Accompanying 6th, 7th, 8th nerve palsy • Crossed hemiplegia • Horner's syndrome
2. Medulla	Ipsilateral hemifacial sensory loss	• Lateral medullary or Wallenberg syndrome • 9th, 10th, 11th, 12th cranial nerve palsy
Preganglionic (prior to gasserian ganglion in Meckel's cave) cerebellopontine angle	Fascial numbness (ipsilateral)	7th, 8th cranial nerve and ipsilateral cerebellar signs
Middle cranial fossa		
1. Gasserian ganglion (Meckel's cave)	Ipsilateral fascial numbness with motor weakness of 5th innervated muscles	Gradenigo syndrome (6th, 7th cranial nerve)
2. Skull base	Ipsilateral fascial numbness and motor weakness	• Headache • Meningeal signs
Cavernous sinus region	Ipsilateral fascial sensory loss (pure sensory) in V1 V2 distribution	• Horner's • 3rd, 6th nerve palsy • Proptosis
Individual branches of trigeminal nerve		
1. Ophthalmic division (V1)	Sensory loss in V1 distribution	Lesion in cavernous sinus or superior orbital fissure
2. Maxillary division (V2)	Sensory loss in V2 distribution	Lesion in maxillary region or Foramen rotundum
3. Mandibular division (V3)	Fascial numbness in V3 distribution with weakness muscles of mastication	Foramen ovale or mandibular region

4.7.5 Localization of 5th Nerve According to Signs

Hemifacial sensory loss	• Supranuclear pathway • Infranuclear from nucleus up to gasserian ganglion (beyond which individual branches are involved)
Hemifacial sensory loss with weakness of masticatory muscles	• Nucleus in pons • Gasserian ganglion in Meckel's cave • Mandibular nerve in Foramen ovale or mandibular region
Isolated touch sensation loss in hemifacial distribution	• Pontine nuclear lesion
Pain and temperature loss in facial distribution with intact touch	Lesion of descending tract of trigeminal up to cervical cord
Onion peel distribution of sensory loss (around lips with a more severe loss around the lips with zones of progressively reducing loss of sensation in an onion peel distribution)	5th sensory nuclear lesion

4.8 Facial Nerve or 7th Cranial Nerve

4.8.1 Neuroanatomy (Figs. 4.26 and 4.27)

1. Motor supply—muscles of facial expression, the scalp and ear and posterior belly of digastric, stylohyoid, stapedius muscle, buccinators, and platysma.
2. Sensory innervation—small area around the concha of the auricle and external auditory canal.
3. Special sensory—taste sensation to anterior 2/3rd of tongue.
4. Parasympathetic:
   (a) Submandibular and sublingual salivary glands
   (b) Nasal, palatine, and pharyngeal mucous glands
   (c) Lacrimal glands

4.8.2 Intracranial Course

The nerve arises in the pons as a large motor root from the motor nucleus in the pons and a smaller sensory root. The motor nucleus receives UMN input from bilateral cerebral hemispheres. The two roots travel together to the internal acoustic meatus (opening in petrous part of temporal bone) along and lateral to the 8th nerve and leave the internal acoustic meatus to enter the facial canal, which has a Z-shaped structure and emerges out from the stylomastoid foramen. Within the facial canal, the two roots join to form the facial nerve. The nerve forms the geniculate ganglion in the facial canal and the facial nerve gives rise to three branches in the facial canal in serial order:

1. Greater petrosal nerve—parasympathetic supply to lacrimal gland.
2. Nerve to stapedius—motor fibers to stapedius muscle of the middle ear.
3. Chorda tympani branch—taste fibers from anterior 2/3 of tongue and parasympathetic supply to submandibular and sublingual glands.

4.8.3 Extracranial Course

The facial nerve exits the facial canal through the stylomastoid foramen and passes forward through the parotid gland. The first branch after exiting out from the stylomastoid foramen is the poste-

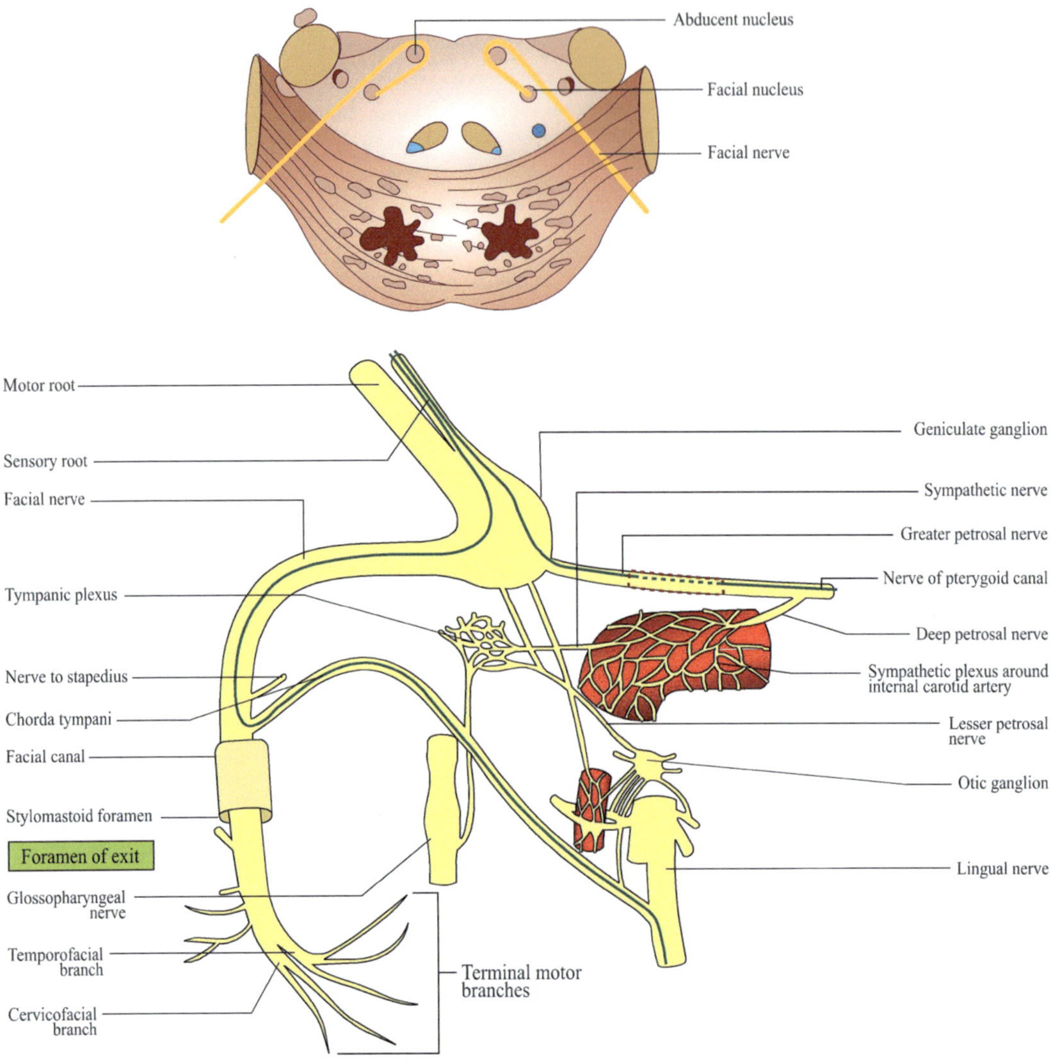

Fig. 4.26 Facial Nerve origin and course

rior auricular nerve, which provides motor supply to the muscles around the ear. The next branch supplies motor innervation to the digastric muscle and stylohyoid muscle. The facial nerve then passes through the parotid gland where it divides into the terminal branches

1. Temporal
2. Zygomatic
3. Buccal
4. Mandibular
5. Cervical branch—supplies the platysma muscle

Interestingly the facial nerve passes through the parotid but does not innervate it. The parotid is supplied by the glossopharyngeal nerve.

4.8.4 Clinical Testing

1. *Motor function*
   (a) *Inspect the face* as a whole, especially for the absence of wrinkles of the forehead or nasolabial fold on the side of paralysis.
   (b) Assess for *spontaneous blinking*—which may be reduced on the paralyzed side.

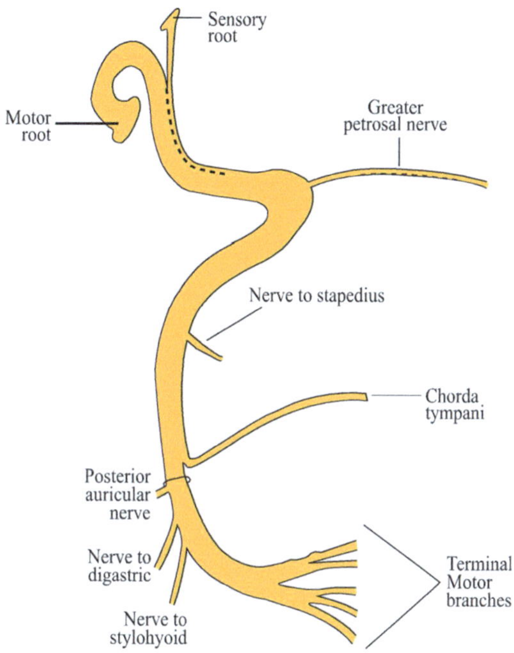

Fig. 4.27 Facial nerve branches

(c) Assess for *emotional movements,* e.g., while smiling. Isolated loss of emotional movements with intact motor function is called Emotional 7th nerve palsy and may occur in lesions of corticobulbar fibers travelling from the contralateral cortex to the thalamus.
(d) Assess for involuntary movements, e.g., dyskinesia's, fasciculations, and hemifacial spasm.
(e) Assess the upper, middle, and lower facial muscles by asking the patient to carry out various motor movements of the face—raise eyebrows, frown, tightly close the eyelids, pinch up the nose, blow cheeks, show teeth by smiling, purse the lips. Examiner can attempt to open the eyelids when the patient is squeezing them or attempt to open the pursed lips.
(f) Platysma is difficult to evaluate but can be evaluated by the patient opening the mouth against resistance or clenching the teeth and looking for contraction of the platysma.
(g) Weakness of the Stapedius muscle can be assessed by evaluating for hyperacusis, especially for low tones.

2. *Examination of taste*
   (a) Explain the test to the patient.
   (b) Patient protrudes the tongue out to one side and keeps it protruded throughout the test. The tongue may be held manually with a piece of gauze and prevented from retraction back into the mouth.
   (c) The examiner touches the lateral side of the tongue about 2 cm from the tip with moistened sugar (for sweet), salt (for salty), vinegar (for sour), and last of all with quinine (for bitter taste that may outlast the stimulus) in that order.
   (d) Patient has to inform by gesture (not talking or taking the tongue in) whether he/she could feel any taste and then should indicate the type of taste by pointing at a written card, which has the types of taste written on it.
   (e) Both sides of the tongue are examined similarly and compared to each other.
3. *Lacrimation and Salivation*
   (a) The flow of tears from both eyes following inhalation of ammonia can be compared. The *Schirmer test* demonstrates the amount of tearing by placing a strip of filter or litmus paper or commercially available strips placed in the inferior conjunctival sac of the lower eyelid and measuring the length of moistening on each side. The length of moisturization is measured in millimeters and compared with normative data.
   (b) Flow of saliva can be assessed by placing few drops of lemon juice on the tongue and asking the patient to raise the tip of the tongue so that the examiner can visualize the flow of saliva.

4.8.5 Upper Motor Facial Palsy (UMN)

- Lesions from frontal cortex up to but not involving the motor nucleus in the pons can result in UMN facial palsy.
- Due to bilateral supranuclear supply to the upper face, the upper part of the face is less affected than the lower half and the patient has

only partial difficulty in closing the eye and the paralysis of the upper facial muscles is significantly milder than involvement of the lower half of the face.

- Emotional 7th nerve palsy due to involvement of the frontal cortex or projections to the thalamus causes only inability to move the facial muscles during emotions, e.g., laughing or crying with near intact motor strength on clinical testing.

4.8.6 Lower Motor Facial Palsy

- Lesion of the facial nucleus in pons, facial nerve in the pons or the facial nerve as it exits from the pons, facial nerve in the CP angle or facial canal or nerve in parotid gland can result in Lower Motor Facial Palsy (LMN) seventh nerve palsy.
- Characteristically the upper part of the face is severely affected with marked difficulty in closing the eyelids. Attempts to close the eyelid leads to the up rolling of the eyeball, which is called the Bell's phenomenon and is seen in LMN facial palsy.

4.8.7 Sites of LMN 7th Palsy

- *Pons (Nuclear)*—infranuclear 7th palsy at this site is usually associated with ipsilateral 6th nerve palsy due to facial nerve winding around the 6th nerve nucleus. There are accompanying contralateral long tract signs.
- *Cerebellopontine region*—5th and 8th cranial nerves also affected along with 7th cranial nerve.
- *Lesion proximal to the Greater Petrosal nerve*—results in loss of lacrimation in the ipsilateral eye (dry eye).
- *Lesion between geniculate ganglion and Nerve to Stapedius*—results in hyperacusis or distortion of sound in the ipsilateral ear, especially for low tones.
- *Facial canal proximal to Chorda Tympani*—loss of taste on the ipsilateral anterior 2/3 of tongue, and ipsilateral loss of salivation and tear production.
- *Lesion distal to Chorda Tympani*—pure motor weakness with no hyperacusis or loss of taste.
- *Lesion in Parotid gland or Face*—pure motor weakness with the involvement of some but not all facial muscles.

4.9 Vestibulocochlear or 8th Cranial Nerve

4.9.1 Neuroanatomy

- The Vestibulocochlear nerve conveys afferents from the cochlear and the vestibular apparatus via the internal auditory meatus to the pontomedullary junction where the cochlear and vestibular nuclei are situated.
- The vestibular component arises from the vestibular nuclei complex in the inferior pons and medulla.
- The cochlear component arises from the ventral and dorsal cochlear nuclei situated in the inferior pons close to the inferior cerebellar peduncle.
- The two vestibular and cochlear components combine in the pons to form the vestibulo–cochlear nerve, which reaches the cerebellopontine angle and exits the cranium via the internal acoustic meatus of the temporal bone where it lies medial to the facial nerve. While traversing the distal part of the internal acoustic meatus, it splits into the vestibular and cochlear nerves. The vestibular nerve innervates the vestibular system of the inner ear involved in balance and the cochlear nerve innervates the spiral ganglia involved in hearing.
- There are bilateral hearing pathways from the cochlear nucleus to the primary auditory cortex (area 41, 42) in the superior temporal gyrus and hence even a complete lesion of one side primary auditory cortex will not result in any significant hearing loss (Figs. 4.28 and 4.29).

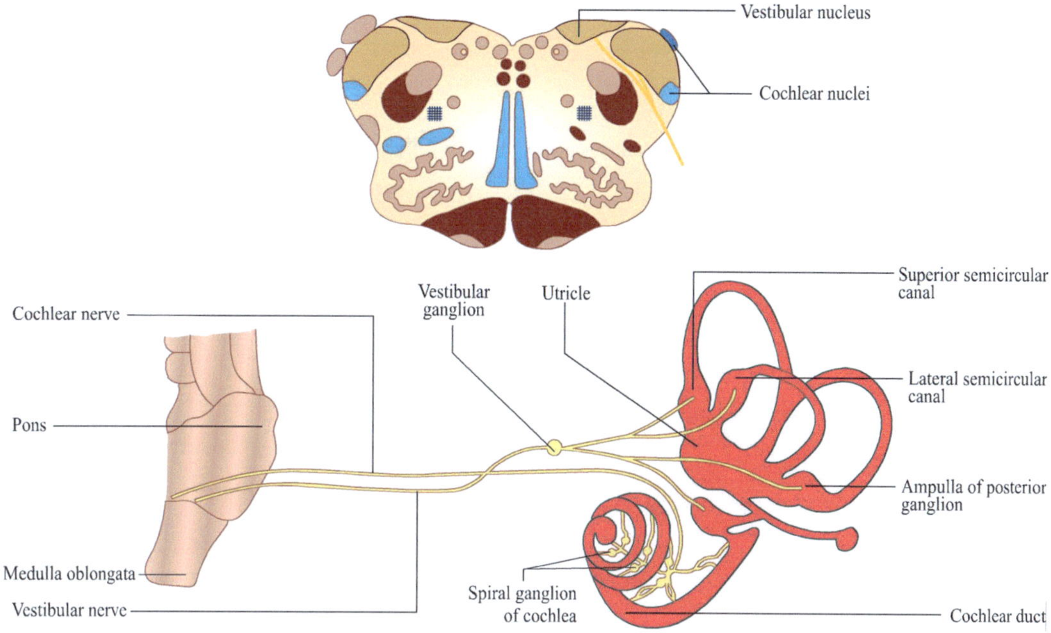

Fig. 4.28 Vestibulo-cocchlear nerve: origin and course

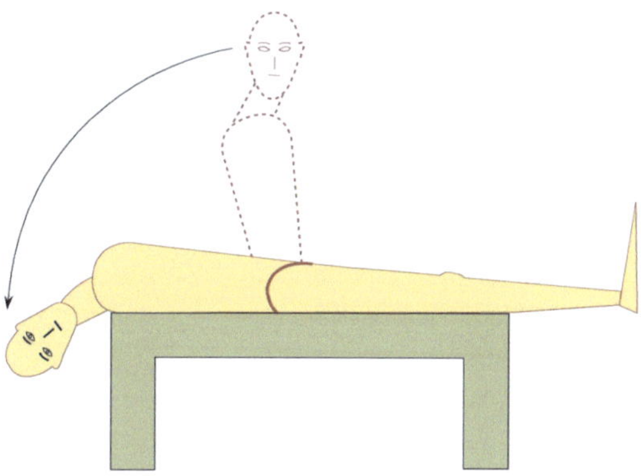

Fig. 4.29 Hallpike's manouevre

4.9.2 Clinical Testing

4.9.2.1 Tests of Cochlear Function

Air conduction of sound to the drum and bony ossicles is the usual method of hearing and is twice as more efficient as the conduction through bone. Conductive deafness results from middle ear dysfunction and inner ear or neural pathway dysfunction result in sensory-neural or perceptive deafness.

1. *Bedside hearing test (Voice test)*
   (a) Test one ear at a time. Sit close to the tested ear in a manner that lip reading is not possible. Mask the opposite ear with a crumpled piece of paper or rubbing the index finger and thumb close to the patient's ear.
   (b) Whisper in the tested ear from a distance of 60 cm (whisper softly the number 26 or 68 to test high tones and 42 or 100 for testing low tones).
   (c) If the patient cannot hear, gradually increase the intensity of sound gradually to normal conversational volume.
   (d) Test the other ear similarly.
2. *Rinne test*
   (a) Use a 512-Hz tuning fork (128 Hz tuning fork is used for testing vibration) and after striking it place it close to the external ear canal with the vibrating prongs toward the meatus (tests Air Conduction or AC). Then place the base of the vibrating tuning fork on the ipsilateral mastoid (for Bone Conduction or BC)

(b) Ask the patient to inform as soon as the bone conduction disappears and immediately place the tuning fork for testing Air conduction. Patient should be able to hear air conduction even when bone conduction has ceased.

(c) Rinne positive = AC > BC (Air conduction is better than bone).

Seen in

(i) Normal Ear

(ii) Sensorineural deafness

(d) Rinne negative = AC < BC

Seen in conductive deafness

3. *Weber test*

(a) The base of the vibrating tuning fork (512 HZ) is held over the center of the forehead and the patient is asked whether the sound is heard over the entire head and both ears equally or only in one ear predominantly.

(b) Weber

(i) Localized to normal ear in: sensorineural deafness

(ii) Localized to abnormal ear in: conductive deafness

4. *Absolute Bone Conduction test*

(a) Bone conduction of the patient by the vibrating tuning fork on the mastoid is compared with that of the examiner—as soon as the patient indicates cessation of sound from the mastoid, place the base of the tuning fork on the mastoid of the examiner to assess whether the sound is still audible despite the patient not being able to hear it.

(b) Normal ABC—normal bone conduction.

Abnormal ABC—reduced bone conduction in sensory neural loss.

5. *Pure Tone Audiometry*

(a) ENT physicians prefer to confirm results of bedside hearing tests with the gold standard audiometry (Pure tone audiometry).

(b) A range of frequencies between 100 and 800 Hz are utilized.

(c) Presence an Air-borne gap of more than 10 db is indicative of conductive deafness.

6. *Loudness Recruitment test*

Under certain situations of unilateral deafness, appreciation of sound of low intensity may be diminished in the affected ear but when the same sound reaches a high intensity it may be heard equally in both ears. This is characteristic of a cochlear dysfunction, e.g., Meniere's disease.

4.9.2.2 Tests of Vestibular Function

1. *Rotational test*

Patient is seated on a rotational chair. For horizontal canals, the head is flexed forward at 30* and for vertical canals it is flexed forward to 120*. The chair is then rotated 10 times in 20 s.

Examine the patient following cessations of the rotation. When rotation has been done to the left, there is nystagmus with slow phase to the left with past pointing and falling to the left.

2. *Caloric test*

Patient lies supine with head flexed 30* for horizontal canals and is requested to fix his/her gaze on an object in front. 50 ml of water is irrigated into the external auditory canal for 45 s, initially 7° below normal temperature (30°) and then 7° above normal (44°). Duration of nystagmus in forward gaze is measured. The test is then repeated on the other side and the results are compared to assess for canal paresis (no response to hot or cold), directional preponderance (reduced response) in same direction. For example, cold water in the left and warm water in right.

3. *Dix-halpike test*

Patient is made to sit on the examination couch and passive neck movements are assessed to be free and painless. Head(chin) is turned 45* toward the side of the test.

The patient is laid back rapidly with head extended over the edge of the bed.

In patients with BPPV, following a latent period there is a torsional nystagmus beating toward the lower ear with vertigo, lasting for 5–30 s and the response fatigues with repetition. The maneuver can be extended to the Epley maneuver to treat the condition where the patients head is rotated 90* to the opposite direction so that the face faces the floor while still lying on the bed and maintaining 30° extension at the neck and patient is kept in this position for 2 minutes. Finally, the patient is slowly brought to the upright sitting position while maintaining the 45° head rotation.

	Conductive deafness	Sensorineural deafness
Rinne test	AC > BC	AC > BC but both reduced
Weber	Lateralized to abnormal ear	Lateralized to normal ear
Audiometry	Loss of low tones	Loss of high tones
Causes	Pathology of external meatus, middle ear, and Eustachian tube, e.g., ASOM, CSOM	*Cochlear lesion* Meniere's disease Otosclerosis Drugs Prolonged exposure to loud sound *Nerve trunk* Cerebello-pontine angle tumors Meningitis *Brainstem* Stroke Tumors

4.9.3 Electronystagmography (ENG)

- Changes in electric field arising from the retinal pigmented epithelium resulting from movement of the eyeball can be measured by electrodes placed around the eye.
- Electrodes placed lateral to the eye and above the bridge of the nose detect electrical activity produced by lateral eyeball movements and electrodes placed above and below the eye detect vertical eyeball movements.
- Electronystagmography enables nystagmus to be measured more precisely compared to a subjective gross visual observation.
- Electronystagmography can also be utilized to observe eyeball movements/nystagmus during other maneuvers, e.g., rotational and caloric testing and by stimulation for evaluating optokinetic nystagmus.

4.10 The Glossopharyngeal (IXth) and Vagus (X) Nerves

4.10.1 Neuroanatomy

Both the nerves are usually evaluated collectively in view of the difficulty in separating the actions of the two nerves.

4.10.2 Function

4.10.2.1 Glossopharyngeal (IX) (Fig. 4.30)

Motor: Stylopharyngeus (loss of function may cause mild lowering of palatal arch).

Parasympathetic: Supply to parotid gland for salivary secretion.

Sensory: Taste of posterior 1/3rd tongue and light touch and pain sensation over pharynx, tonsillar region, soft palate and middle ear, posterior wall of external auditory canal, and posterior part of tympanic membrane.

1. Glossopharyngeal nerve lesions result in:
   (a) Impaired swallowing.
   (b) Impaired taste sensation over posterior 1/3rd tongue.
   (c) Impaired light touch and pain sensation over pharynx, tonsillar region, soft palate and middle ear, posterior wall of external auditory canal, and posterior part of tympanic membrane.
   (d) Absent gag reflex- on ipsilateral stimulation with preserved gag reflex on contralateral stimulation.

4.10.2.2 Vagus (X) (Figs. 4.31 and 4.32)

Motor:

1. ALL muscles of palate, pharynx, larynx (via recurrent laryngeal nerve) except tensor velli palitini (5th nerve), mylohyoid (5th nerve), stylohyoid (7th nerve), stylopharyngeus (9th nerve).
2. Motor supply to one tongue muscle (palatoglossus).

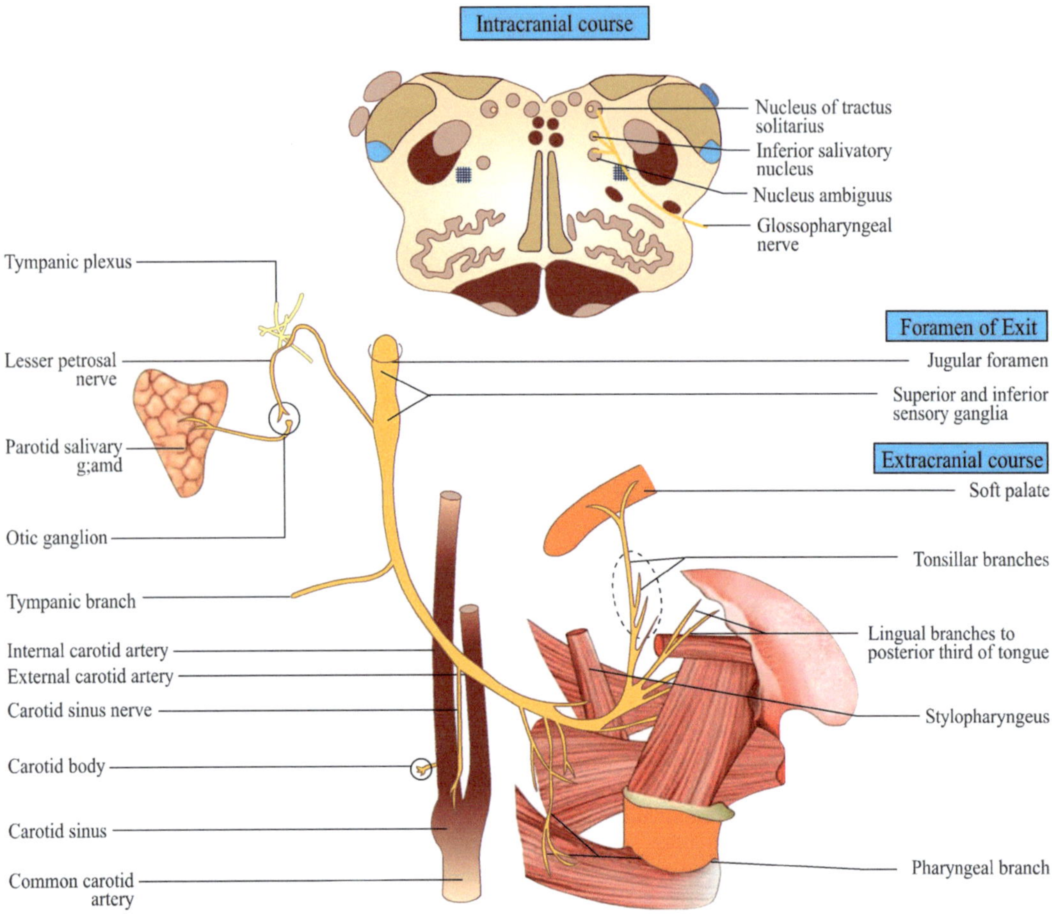

Fig. 4.30 Glossopharyngeal nerve: origin and course

Fig. 4.31 Vagus nerve: origin

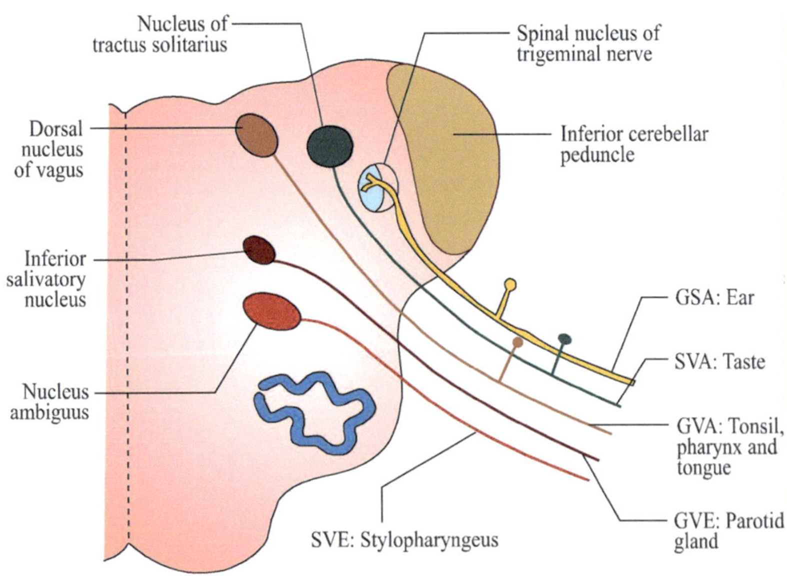

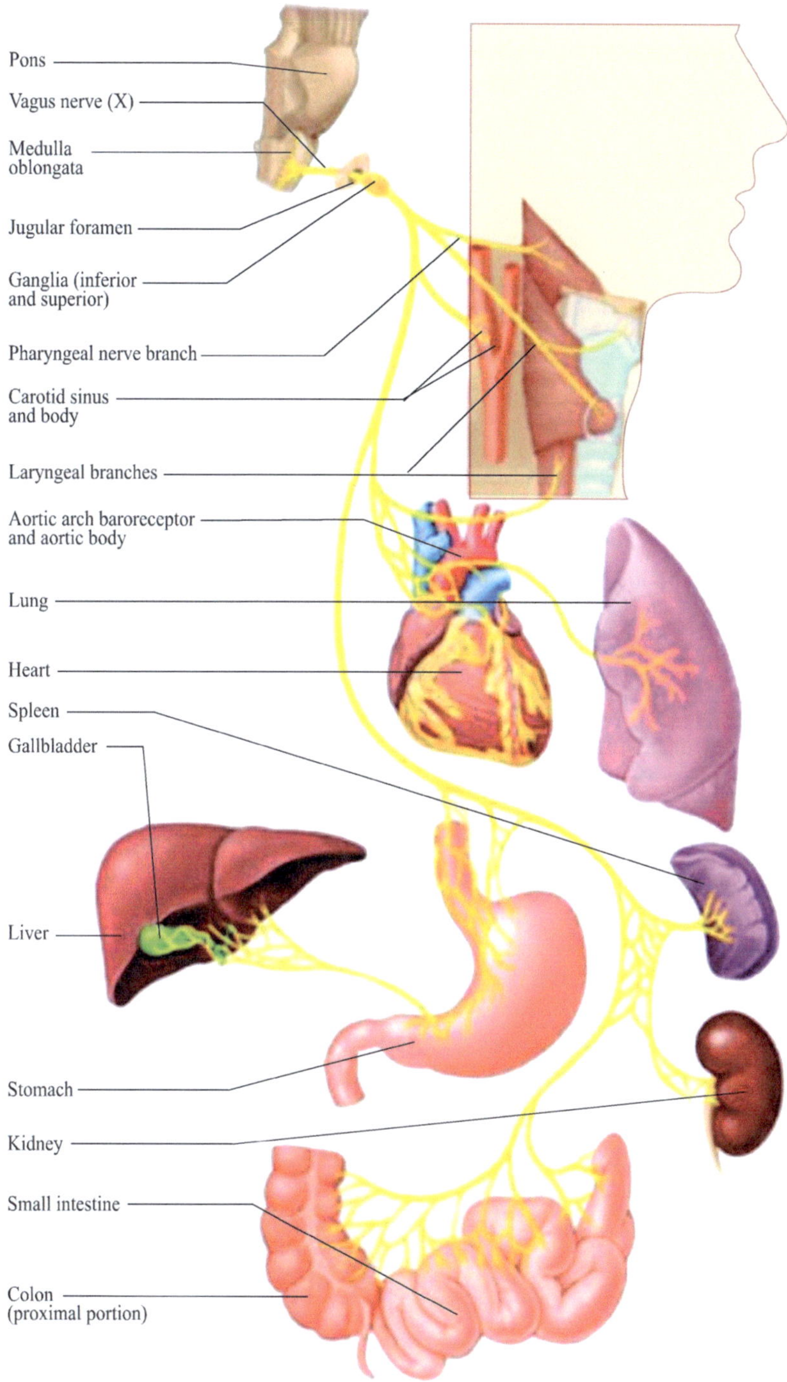

Fig. 4.32 Vagus nerve: origin and branches

Autonomic: Afferents from carotid baroreceptors, parasympathetic supply to and from thorax and abdomen. It is the longest parasympathetic nerve in the body and vagal stimulation can lead to bradycardia, bronchoconstriction, hypotension, increased peristalsis, gastric and intestinal secretions, and inhibition of adrenal function.

Sensory: Pain, temperature and light touch sensation over pharynx, larynx, tympanic membrane, external auditory canal and external ear, and dura mater of posterior fossa.

1. Vagus nerve lesions will result in:
   (a) Palatal weakness
   (b) Pharyngeal weakness
   (c) Laryngeal weakness
   (d) Abnormality of esophageal motility, gastric acid secretion, gall bladder emptying and abnormalities of heart rate, and other autonomic dysfunction.

The glossopharyngeal nerve originates from the nucleus ambiguous in the medulla and nerve rootlets emerge from the medulla just rostral to those of the vagus nerve. It then leaves the cranial cavity through the jugular foramen and descends into the neck where it provides branches to the stylopharyngeus and sensation to the carotid sinus and body and terminates in the pharynx by giving the terminal branches—lingual, pharyngeal, and tonsils.

The vagus nerve emerges from the medulla just below the glossopharyngeal nerve and exits the cranial cavity along with the glossopharyngeal nerve through the jugular foramen. Then it passes into the carotid sheath between the internal carotid artery and the internal jugular vein into the neck, chest, and abdomen where it contributes to innervation of the viscera down up to the colon.

4.10.3 Clinical Testing

1. *Motor function*
   (a) Look for nasal twang (palatal dysfunction), bovine (weak) cough, nasal regurgitation of saliva, hoarse voice (laryngeal palsy).
   (b) Ask the patient to open the mouth wide and allow a little time to allow the tongue to rest on the floor (preferable without the use of tongue depressor).
   (c) Look for symmetry of bilateral palatal arches and for central position of the uvula.
   (d) Ask the patient to say a loud "ahh" and evaluate for:
      (i) Pharyngeal curtain movement—bilateral symmetrical
      (ii) Elevation of both palatal arches, symmetrically
      (iii) Uvula rises up but remains central
   (e) Look for:
      (i) Unilateral loss of pharyngeal curtain movement, loss of palatal elevation, and uvula being pulled to opposite direction by the normal muscle indicating unilateral 9th and 10th palsy.
      (ii) Bilateral restricted pharyngeal and palatal movement with central uvula (bilateral 9th and 10th palsy).
2. Sensory function
   (a) Touch—throat swab with cotton wool safely attached can be used to evaluate touch sensation on posterior 1/3 tongue, palate, pharynx, and tonsillar region.
   (b) Taste—it is difficult to evaluate taste sensation on the posterior 1/3 of the tongue and a galvanic stimulation current of 2–4 mA can be used to produce a metallic taste and is compared on both sides. Alternatively, a quinine soaked cotton bud may be applied to the posterior third of the tongue and the patient should be able to feel the bitter taste without speaking or moving the tongue.
3. Gag reflex
   Afferent—glossopharyngeal
   Efferent—vagus
   (a) Touch the pharyngeal wall behind the pillars of the fauces with a throat swab. Patient can compare the quality of touch

on both sides and each side stimulation will result in gagging (contraction of the pharynx, palate, and elevation of the uvula).

Unilateral 9th nerve lesion Stimulation on the paralyzed side will not be felt by the patient and gag reflex will not occur on stimulating on the paralyzed side. However, stimulation of the normal side will produce a normal gag on the paralyzed side. Isolated lesions of the 9th nerve are rare.

Unilateral 10th nerve lesion

- Patient will appreciate sensation on either side.
- Stimulation of either side will not produce elevation of the palate arch on the paralyzed side. Stimulation on the paralyzed side will, however, result in contraction of the opposite palatal arch.

Lesions of superior laryngeal nerve
This is a predominantly sensory nerve with motor supply only to the cricothyroid muscle.

Lesion of the superior laryngeal nerve may cause mild hoarseness of voice.

Lesion of recurrent laryngeal nerve
This has a long intrathoracic course—left nerve has a longer course than the right nerve and provides motor supply to all the muscles of the larynx except the cricothyroid (supplied by the superior laryngeal nerve).

Unilateral lesion of recurrent laryngeal nerve
Mild-to-moderate hoarseness of voice.

Paralyzed cord lies in midline with failure to abduct.

Bilateral lesion of recurrent laryngeal nerve
Severe hoarseness and stridor with respiratory compromise

Both cords lie approximately in midline with failure to abduct.

4.11 Spinal Accessory Nerve: 11th Cranial Nerve

4.11.1 Neuroanatomy

The accessory nerve has 2 parts—the cranial and the spinal accessory parts. The *Cranial accessory* is formed from nerve fibers from the nucleus ambiguous and then soon leaves the accessory nerve to rejoin the vagus nerve and cannot be examined separately.

The *Spinal accessory* is the component that is clinically evaluated and the nerve fibers arise from the cervical spinal cord C2–6 segments and these roots pass rostrally up into the medulla and emerge as the spinal accessory nerve. It travels along the IX and X cranial nerves through the jugular foramen and supplies motor supply to the sternocleidomastoid and upper part of the trapezius muscle (Fig. 4.33).

4.11.2 Clinical Testing

1. Sternocleidomastoid
   (a) The sternocleidomastoid flexes the head toward the ipsilateral shoulder and rotates the occiput toward the ipsilateral shoulder and the face or chin to the opposite side shoulder.
   (b) Both sternocleidomastoid muscles contracting together pull the head forward and downward.
   (c) Ask the patient to turn his/her head to one side and resist the movement by placing your hand on the face. Feel the contraction of the opposite side sternocleidomastoid. For example, left sternocleidomastoid examined with turning the head to the right.
   (d) Ask the patient to push against your hand placed on the forehead. Can check contraction of bilateral sternocleidomastoid with this procedure. Inspect and palpate the contraction of the muscles.

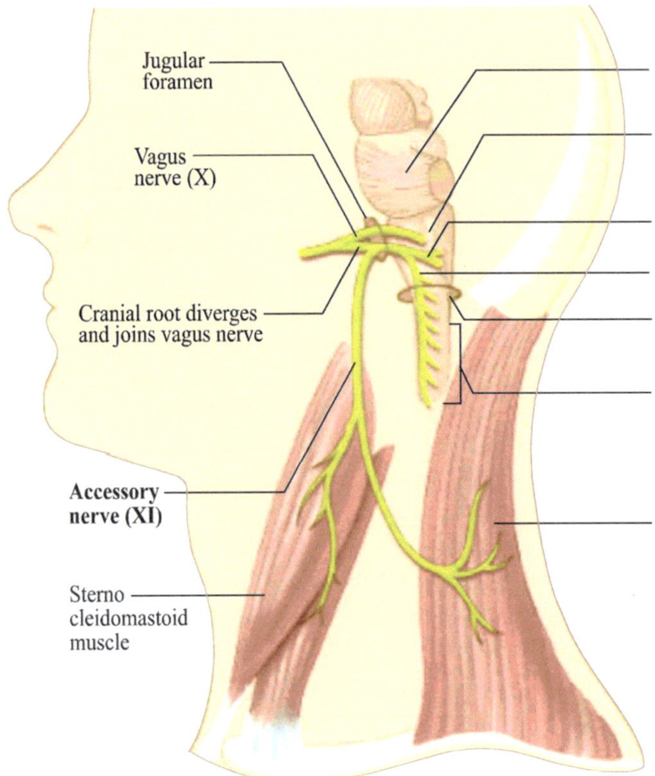

Fig. 4.33 Accesory nerve course

2. *Trapezius*
   (a) The trapezius retracts the head and draws it ipsilaterally and elevates, retracts, and rotates the scapula and hence assists in abducting the arm above horizontal.
   (b) In paralysis of the Trapezius observe for drooping of the shoulder and flattening of the trapezius ridge and wasting of the muscle. The upper part of the scapula moves laterally and the inferior end of the scapula moves inward.
   (c) Ask the patient to shrug the shoulder or push the shoulder up while the examiner attempts to push the shoulder downward. Even feeble individuals will not allow the shoulder to fall by pressure exerted by the examiner.

Bilateral sternocleidomastoid lesion

1. Head falls backward
2. Seen in
   (a) Motor neuron disease
   (b) Muscular dystrophies

Bilateral trapezius weakness

- Inability to shrug the shoulder and head falls forward.

Unilateral sternocleidomastoid weakness

- Fail to turn the head against resistance to the opposite side.

4.12 The Hypoglossal Nerve or XIIth Cranial Nerve

4.12.1 Neuroanatomy

The 12th nerve arises from hypoglossal nucleus in the medulla as a number of rootlets that emerge from the front of the medulla in the anterolateral sulcus, which separates the olive and the pyramid. The nerve passes through the subarachnoid space and pierces the dura mater near the hypoglossal canal which is an opening in the occipital bone of the skull. After emerging from the hypoglossal canal it gives off a meningeal branch and picks up a branch from the anterior ramus of C1. The 12th nerve then travels along the vagus and the accessory nerve and passes between the internal carotid artery and internal jugular vein to supply the extrinsic and intrinsic tongue muscles.

The hypoglossal nerve supplies all the extrinsic and intrinsic tongue muscles except for palatoglossus (Innervated by vagus).

1. *Extrinsic muscles*
   - Paired Genioglossus, styloglossus, hyoglossus, and chondroglossus.
   - Extrinsic muscles pass from skull or hyoid bone to the tongue and serve to protrude and retract the tongue and move the root up and down.
2. *Intrinsic muscles*
   - Superior and inferior longitudinalis, transversus, and verticalis.
   - These intrinsic muscles both arise and end within the tongue and aid in changing the length, width, and curvature of the dorsal surface of the tongue and turn the non-protruded tongue from side to side (Fig. 4.34).

4.12.2 Clinical Testing

- Request the patient to open the mouth and observe the tongue in a *resting position* for surface, size, shape, and position. Look for any atrophy that will be seen as prominent

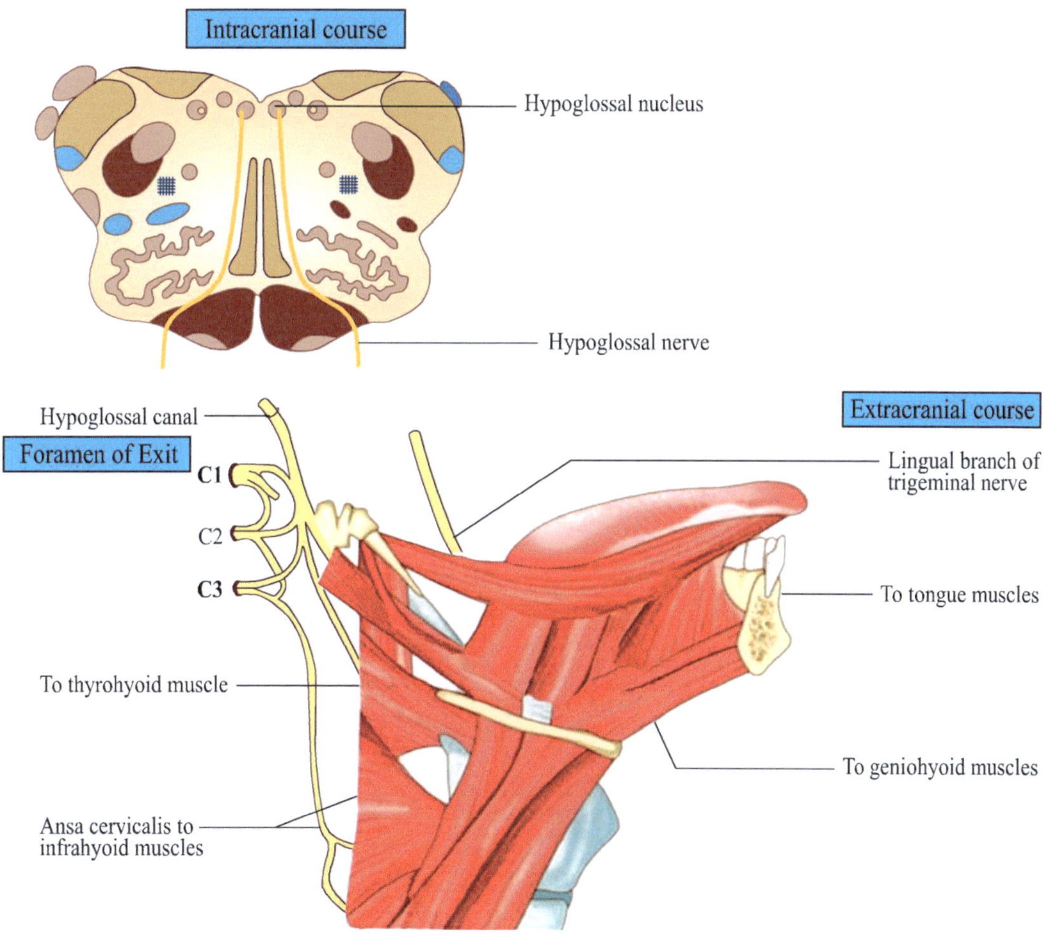

Fig. 4.34 Hypoglossal nerve: origin and course

longitudinal folds and loss of bulk. Hypertrophy of the tongue may be seen in Down's syndrome, Infantile hypothyroidism, Acromegaly, or Amyloidosis. Look for abnormal movement, especially fasciculation.

- Request the patient to protrude the tongue and request to bring it out straight. One can compare deviation of the tongue by comparing the tip of the tongue to the center point between the lower 2 incisors. One can assess power by asking the patient to push the examiner's fingers through the cheek and compare the extent of push on the finger on both sides.
- Ask the patient to rapidly move the tongue side to side and up and down and observe for the speed of movement. In spastic tongue (UMN lesions) movements are slow and difficult with maintained shape and bulk.
- Tongue deviated to: pushed by the normal side
- One side: toward the paralyzed side
- Atrophy of half of tongue
  - Wasted, Ipsilateral
  - LMN12th nerve lesion
- Small, atrophic, bilateral tongue with inability to protrude and fasciculations—Bilateral 12th N palsy (bulbar palsy)
- Stiff, normal, or small-sized tongue with inability to protrude
  - Bilateral UMN palsy
  - Pseudobulbar palsy
- Alternate protrusion and retraction (Jack in the box)—Chorea
- Tapping the tongue will cause a dent, which disappears immediately, and prolonged persistence of the dent is seen in Myotonia.

5 Examination of Speech

Speech disorders fall into three broad categories:

(A) *Language disorders*
Dysphasia or aphasia
(B) *Difficulty in enunciation* or pronunciation
Dysarthria or anarthria
(C) *Disorders of volume* of speech
Dysphonia
(D) *Mutism*
Mutism is a disorder of conciousness rather than a speech disorder. Conscious patient but makes no attempt to speak or produce sound even though has the ability to produce speech. Most of these patients of akinetic mute state have paucity of thought, action, and speech even though the ability for these modalities is preserved.

5.1 Language Disorders or Aphasia

Assessment of language involves evaluating:

(a) Spontaneous speech (fluency, word output)
(b) Comprehension
(c) Repetition
(d) Paraphasia
(e) Reading
(f) Writing

5.1.1 Spontaneous Speech

- Check for fluency vs nonfluency. Patient's spontaneous word output in the course of a conversation and in response to general questions is judged. Patient is asked open-ended questions, e.g., "why are you in hospital" or "what do you do on a typical day at home or office."
- In nonfluent speech patients will produce <50 words/minute with shortened phrase lengths and production of speech is effortful and the patient may use telegraphic speech with loss of melody (prosody).
- *Anatomical Substitute* for fluency–Nonfluency indicates damage to frontal lobe language region anterior to the fissure of Rolando (central sulcus), especially the Broca's area (posterior part of inferior frontal gyrus, area 44) and hence is also labelled as *anterior aphasia*.

5.1.2 Comprehension of Speech

1. An initial judgment of auditory comprehension can be determined in the course of normal conversation.
2. Can conduct specific tests for assessing comprehension:
   (a) *Commands*—One step part body command (show your tongue) or multiple step

V. Suri, *Clinical Neurological Examination and Localization*,
https://doi.org/10.1007/978-981-16-1228-2_5

commands (open your right hand, and then touch the right-hand index figure to the tip of your nose).

(b) *Yes/No responses*—Patient is asked questions where they have to answer yes or no, e.g.:

Is your name Mr. Sharma?
Is sugar sweet?
Is New Delhi in India?

(c) *Pointing responses*—Patient has to comprehend the command and gesticulate accordingly, e.g.:

I. Point to the fan
II. Point to my pen
III. Point to the source of illumination in the room (complex)

Anatomical substrate for comprehension

Comprehension is impaired with damage to the temporoparietal language regions posterior to the fissure of Ronaldo (central sulcus), especially the Wernicke's area (posterior part of superior temporal gyrus area 22) and is hence also labelled as *posterior aphasia.*

5.1.3 Repetition

Patient is asked to repeat simple and complex sentences and some rich in grammatical words, e.g., "No ifs and or buts."

Anatomical substrate

(i) *Perisylvian localization:* In most patients repetition is impaired and the impairment parallels other defects in spoken languages.

(ii) *Conduction aphasia*: Repetition impairment is severe and the sole abnormality. This is caused by lesions of the Arcuate fibers connecting the Broca's with the Wernicke's area. Patients can verbalize fluently with relatively intact comprehension but cannot repeat, e.g., a soldier tried several times to repeat the sentence "this is a rifle" and after several failed attempts says…

"……. Oh hell …. I know it is a gun"

(iii) *Extrasylvian localization* repetition may be significantly preserved despite other language deficits.

Transcortical motor aphasia (TCM)—Nonfluent speech but fluent repetition.

Transcortical sensory aphasia (TCS)—Impaired comprehension but preserved repetition result in patients repeating sentences spoken by the examiner—pallilalia.

5.1.4 Paraphasic Errors

Substitution of intended words with incorrect words is called paraphasia. They are of 3 types:

(i) *Literal or phonemic paraphasia*

A part of the word is misspoken,

For example, orange becomes torange or orancel.

(ii) *Verbal or global paraphasia*

When an entire word is substituted.

For example, orange becomes banana or car.

Semantic paraphasia is where the entire word is substituted but within the same family. For example, orange becomes lemon.

(iii) *Neologistic paraphasia*

Where entirely novel word is created, e.g, Orange becomes rafontin.

Anatomic substrate—paraphasic errors can occur with lesions anywhere within the language system and do not carry anatomic implications. Usually, phonemic paraphasias are more common in anterior aphasia and global neologistic paraphasias are more common in posterior aphasias.

5.1.5 Naming: Word Finding Difficulty (Anomia)

Difficulty in naming is almost invariable in all aphasic patients. Patients with predominant word finding difficulty will have circumlocution (talk around words). It can be evaluated by:

(i) *Confrontation naming*—patient is asked to name common objects in the room, body parts, and colors pointed by the examiner.
(ii) *Word list generation*—patients are asked to provide a list.

For example, names of animals, words starting with the letter "A." A normal response can elicit up to >12 names per minute.

5.1.6 Reading (Alexia)

In most cases of aphasia, reading and writing deficits parallel the oral language deficit. However, isolated reading and writing impairment can occur with preserved oral language function.

- Patients are asked to read sentences aloud and assess errors in reading.
- Patients are asked to read and then comprehend the written matter and then perform the written commands. For example, touch your nose with your hand.

5.1.7 Writing (Agraphia)

Patients are asked to write single letters, words, and sentences by writing spontaneous sentences and copying written paragraphs for testing repetition.

For localization purposes, aphasias are characterized into 2 subtypes:

(a) Anterior or posterior (to fissure of Rolando)
(b) Perisylvian (around the sylvian fissure) and Extrasylvian (away from sylvian fissure

	Anterior	Posterior
Spontaneous speech	Nonfluent	Fluent
Comprehension	Preserved	Impaired
Paraphasias	Literal	Verbal Neologistic
Repetition	Preserved in Extrasylvian Impaired in perisylvian	Preserved in Extrasylvian Impaired in perisylvian

	Perisylvian	Extrasylvian
Types	Brocas Conduction Wernke's	Transcortical motor Transcortical sensory
Repetition	Impaired	Preserved

1. *Subcortical Aphasia Syndromes*
   (a) *Striatal–Capsular Aphasia* —may resemble transcortical motor aphasia with nonfluent speech with intact comprehension with relatively intact repetition. Lesions involving dominant putamen, caudate, anterior limb of the internal capsule, and rostral periventricular white matter may result in this impairment.
   (b) *Thalamic Aphasia*—may resemble transcortical sensory aphasia with fluent output, impaired comprehension, and preserved repetition with impaired naming.
2. *Alexia without aphasia (Pure alexia)*

   Oral language (fluency and comprehension) is preserved and also writing. Reading, however, is severely impaired. Patients usually have a painstaking letter-by-letter reading strategy. Usually caused by lesion of the dominant occipital lobe with involvement of selenium of corpus callosum.
3. *Alexia with agraphia*
   (a) Well preserved oral language (fluency and comprehension) with impaired reading and writing.
   (b) Caused from lesion of dominant inferior parietal lobe (angular and supramarginal syrups).
4. *Pure word deafness*—fluent speech with impaired comprehension and repetition. However, unlike Wernicke aphasia these patients have intact comprehension of written material and have no paraphasias.

   It is caused by lesions disconnecting the Wernike's area from the primary auditory area.
5. *Aprosodia*
   (a) Loss of prosody, i.e., loss of melody, rhythm, and timber of speech.
   (b) Usually occurs more commonly with lesions of the speech area of the nondominant hemisphere.

Types of aphasia

Aphasia	Fluency	Comprehension	Repetition	Naming
Global	Abn	Abn	Abn	Abn
Broca	*Abn*	N	Abn	Abn
Conduction	N	N	*Abn*	N
Wernicke's	N	*Abn*	Abn	Abn
Transcortical motor	Abn	N	*N*	Abn
Transcortical sensory	N	Abn	*N* echolalia	Abn
Anomic	N	N	N	*Abn*

N Normal, *Abn* Abnormal

A Fluency

1. Loss in lesions anterior to the central sulcus and preserved in lesions posterior to the central sulcus.
   (a) Nonfluent Anterior aphasia/Broca aphasia
       lesion of posterior inferior frontal lobe or Broca's
       area (area 44).
   (b) Fluent posterior temporal and parietal lobe.

B Comprehension

1. Loss in lesions posterior to the central sulcus and intact in lesions anterior to the central sulcus.
   (a) Poor Comprehension—posterior temporal lesion involving Wernicke's area (area 22).
   (b) Good comprehension—posterior frontal (Broca's)

C Repetition

1. Good repetition: Lesions outside the perisylvian region (Transcortical motor and transcortical sensory)
2. Poor repetition Perisylvian syndrome (Broca's, Wernicke's, Conduction) (Figs. 5.1, 5.2 and 5.3)

5.2 Dysarthria

Impaired articulation or enunciation or pronunciation may occur when there is impaired function of the tongue, lips, palate, larynx, and muscles of respiration on account of an UMN or LMN lesion or there is impairment of the coordinating influence of the extrapyramidal or cerebellar system on these muscles or involvement of the muscles involved directly in speech.

5.2.1 Clinical Evaluation

(a) Assess the speech while patient narrates the history.
(b) Ask the patient to repeat certain phrases, e.g., "baby hippo (predominantly labials)," "yellow lorry" (predominantly linguals), "British constitution" (requiring cerebellar coordination).
(c) Ask the patient to read a paragraph or count till 50.

Notice if the words slur, whether rhythm is jerky, monotonous, or explosive, whether certain letters are not articulated properly, e.g., labials, lingual, gutturals, and whether there is hypernasality.

Types of Dysarthria

1. *Spastic dysarthria*—patient speaks with reduced excursion of the mouth as if talking with a sore tongue or from the back of the throat. Caused by bilateral UMN lesion—pseudo-bulbar palsy. The jaw jerk and gag reflex are usually exaggerated.
2. *Rigid dysarthria*—monotonous voice with disappearance of the accent and words running into one another with a low volume of

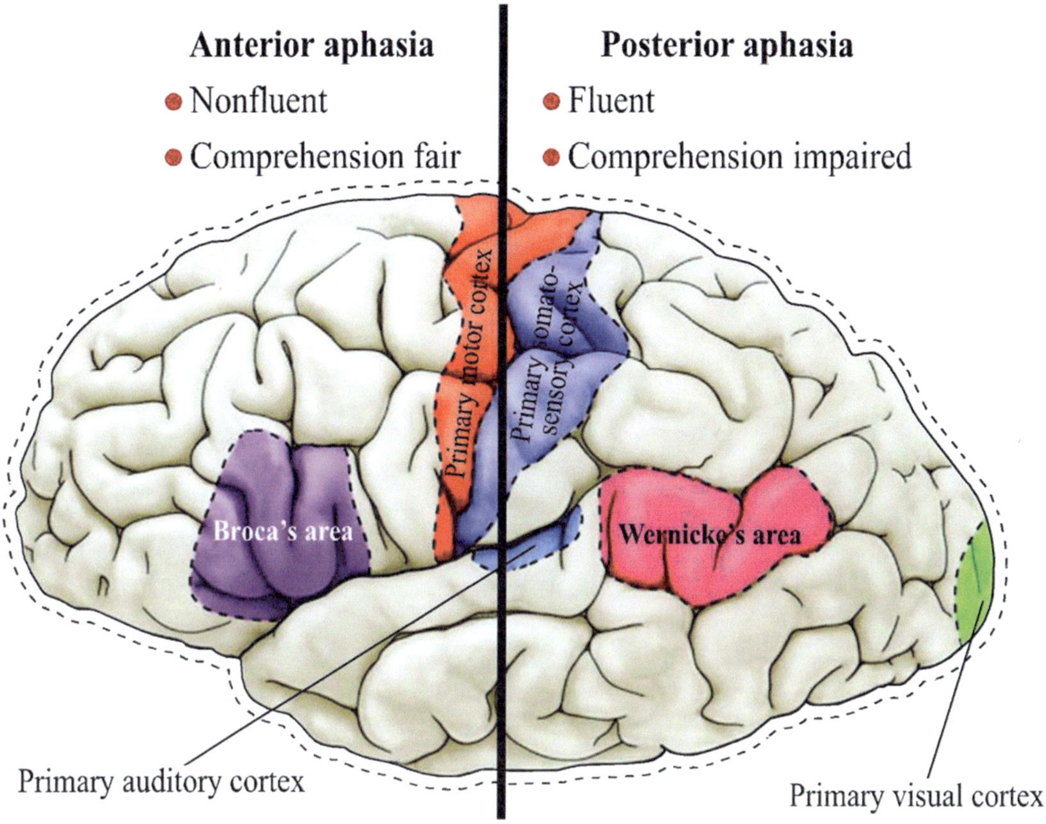

Fig. 5.1 Aphasia: Anterior vs Posterior

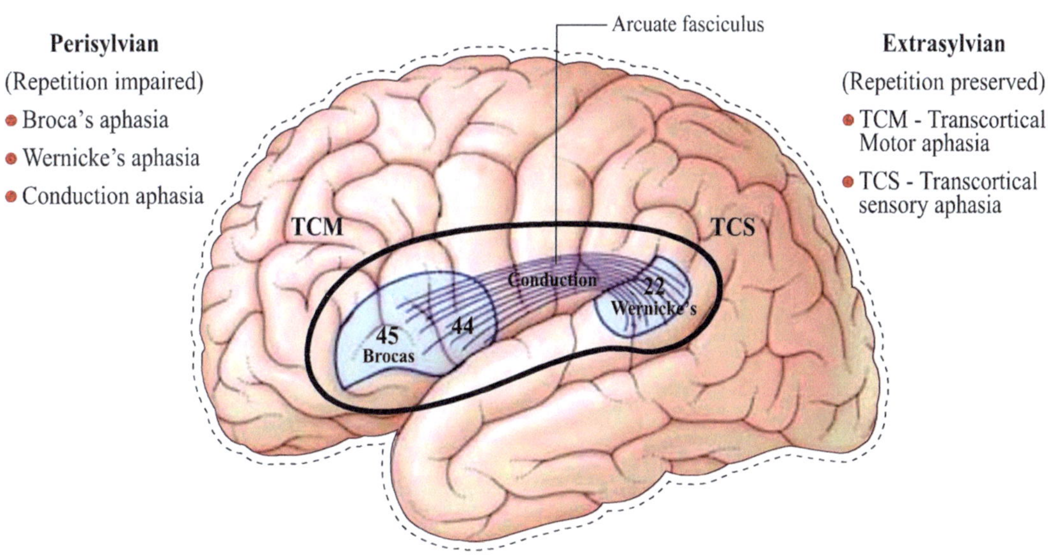

Fig. 5.2 Aphasia: perisylvian vs extra sylvian

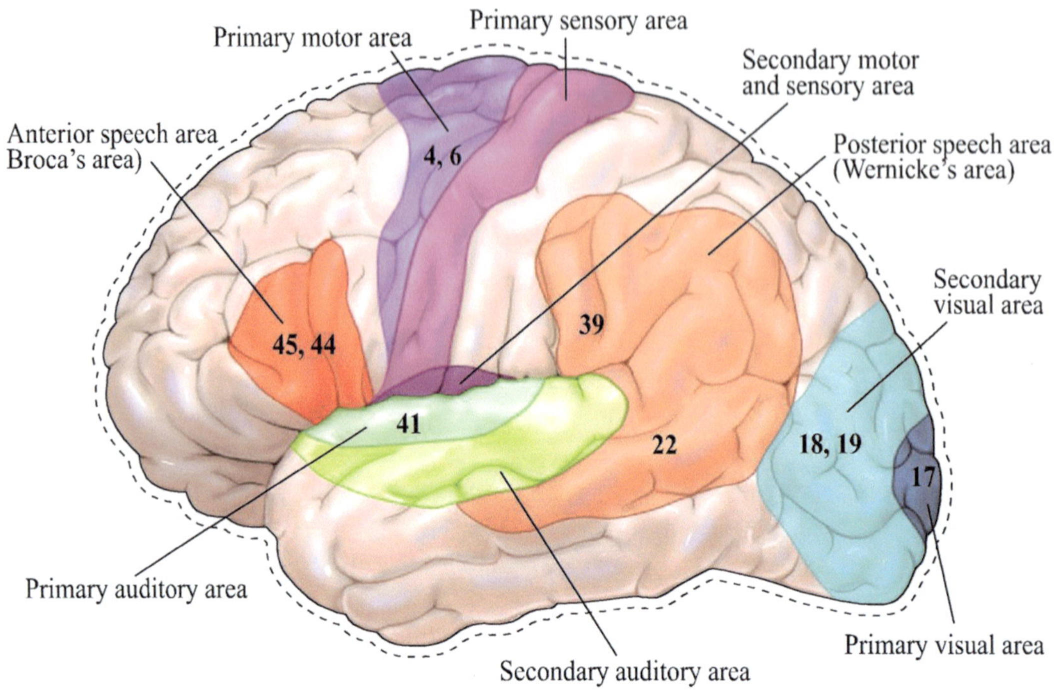

Fig. 5.3 Eloquent areas

speech. Excursions of the tongue and lips are severely reduced. This usually results from extrapyramidal lesions.

3. *Ataxic dysarthria*—slurred and drunken speech which is too soft or too explosive on different letters with words running into one another.
4. Caused by cerebellar or cerebellar connection lesions.
5. *Dysarthria due to lesions of lower motor neuron*
   (a) *Facial muscle* weakness causes difficulty in articulating labials (b, p, m, w) and difficulty in expressing the phrase "baby hippo."
   (b) *Lingual weakness* of tongue muscles will cause difficulty in articulating linguals (y, r, l, v, t, s, x, z) with difficulty in expressing the phrase "yellow lorry."
   (c) *Palatal weakness* will result in hyper nasality and difficulty in expressing words, e.g., "gh" and words like "egg" become "ennngh."
6. *Dysarthria due to neuromuscular junction defect*

True fatigue of speech with slurring becoming prominent after prolonged speaking or while eating food is seen in patients with myasthenia gravis. It can be demonstrated by asking the patient to count till 100 and an initial near normal speech becomes progressively worse with slurring with or without hyper nasality during the latter part of the counting.

5.3 Dysphonia

Dysphonia constitutes disorders of *volume* of speech. Patients speak in reduced volume, which can be reduced to a gentle whisper.

Evaluate the patient by assessing spontaneous speech or by asking the patient to count till 50 and asking the patient to cough forcefully.

Dysphonia may occur in Extrapyramidal disorders or in patients with laryngeal and vocal cord pathology.

6 Motor System Examination

Motor system examination is an extremely important part of the neurological assessment for localization of the site of lesions. Motor system examination provides a pattern of neurological involvement (hemiplegic, quadriplegic, paraplegia, proximal muscles, distal limb weakness in polyneuropathy, or single nerve distribution) (Fig. 6.1).

1. Upper motor neuron lesion

   UMN lesion may arise from lesions affecting the cerebral cortex, corona radiata, basal ganglion, internal capsule, thalamus, brainstem, or spinal cord.

	UMN lesion	LMN lesion
Tone	Spasticity (clasp knife pattern)	Hypotonia
Superficial reflex	Absent	Absent
Deep tendon reflex	Brisk	Absent
Wasting	Mild or none	Moderate to severe
Fasciculation	Not observed	Positive, especially prominent in anterior horn cell disease

UMN lesion from cortex to brainstem (prior to medullary decussation of corticospinal tracts) will present with contralateral UMN hemiplegia accompanied with other characteristic signs according to the site of the lesion.

Cortex	Nondense contralateral hemiplegia with cortical signs, e.g., aphasia, apraxia, agnosia, seizures, and cortical sensory
Corona radiata	Nondense contralateral hemiplegia, absent cortical signs
Internal capsule	Dense contralateral hemiplegia, no cortical signs
Thalamus	Contralateral hemiplegia, ataxic hemiparesis, contralateral hemisensory deficit, or hyperesthesia
BRAINSTEM	• Crossed hemiplegia (ipsilateral cranial nerves and contralateral hemiplegia) • "company they keep"—Localise by adjacent structures involved
Midbrain	Contralateral hemiplegia with ipsilateral 3rd or 4th cranial N palsy
Pons	Contralateral hemiplegia with ipsilateral 6th and 7th N palsy
Medulla	Lateral medulla—ipsilateral cerebellar, ipsilateral 9, 10 cranial nerve palsy and contralateral pain and temperature loss Medial medulla—contralateral hemiplegia, ipsilateral LMN 12th palsy with ipsilateral loss of joint position and vibration sensation (medial lemniscus)

(a) UMN lesions involving the *cord* can result in:
   I. Quadriplegia—when involving cervical segments of the cord.
   II. Paraplegia—when cord pathology involves the cord below T1 segment.

V. Suri, *Clinical Neurological Examination and Localization*,
https://doi.org/10.1007/978-981-16-1228-2_6

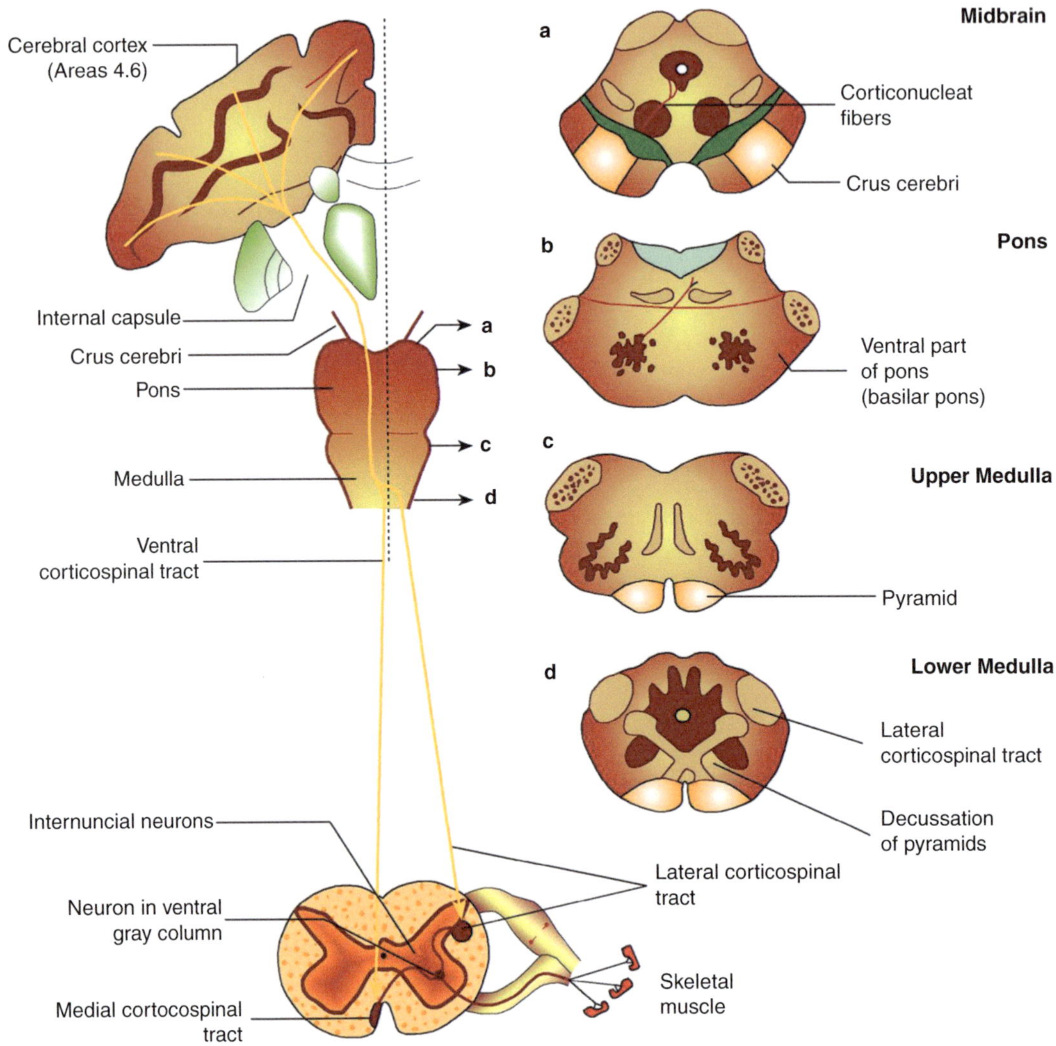

Fig. 6.1 Corticospinal tract: origin and course

III. Hemicord or Brown-Sequard syndrome—when there is an incomplete lesion of the cord (hemicord section).

(b) Ipsilateral UMN motor weakness below the lesion.
(c) Ipsilateral loss of posterior column (light touch, vibration, joint position) below lesion.
(d) Contralateral loss of pain and temperature below the lesion.
(e) Contralateral hyperesthetic area or ipsilateral LMN lesion at the site of lesion.

2. *Lower motor Neuron lesions* may occur due to pathology ranging from the anterior horn cell to nerve (anterior horn cell, motor root, plexus, nerves).

Anterior horn cell	(i) Radicular distribution of motor weakness (ii) Prominent fasciculations (iii) Prominent wasting
Root	(i) Motor and sensory loss in the distribution of radicles (ii) May have a pure motor or mixed sensor motor pattern
Plexus	Multiple nerves originating from the plexus are involved Usually unilateral findings
Nerve	(i) Single nerve distribution (ii) Mononeuritis multiplex distribution (multiple noncontiguous nerves) (iii) Polyneuropathy (length dependent, glove, and stocking) distribution (iv) Usually both sensory and motor involvement

3. Mixed UMN and LMN involvement is seen in:
   (a) Motor neuron disease
   (b) Myeloradiculopathy, e.g., subacute combined degeneration of the cord (SACD), syrinx, cord tumors, myeloradiculopathy from arachnoiditis.
4. Neuromuscular junction
   Usually characterized by:
   a. True fatigability—repeated activity results in progressive weakness
   b. Pure motor involvement
   c. Select group of muscles, e.g., ocular (ptosis with failure to squeeze close eye and ocular muscles involvement), bulbar, and proximal muscles.
5. Muscle disorders
   Involvement is usually characterized by:
   (a) Pure motor involvement
   (b) Select group of muscles, e.g., in fasicoscapulo humero or predominately proximal muscles.
   (c) Wasting usually less prominent.
   (d) Deep tendon reflexes are usually preserved (proportionate to motor power preservation).
   (e) Associated pseudohypertrophy of muscles.
   (f) Tenderness of muscles with dysphagia and neck extensor weakness seen in inflammatory polymyositis.

Clinical Assessment of the MOTOR SYSTEM includes:

1. Inspection for Bulk
   (a) Abnormal movements
   (b) Contractures
2. Assessment of TONE
3. Assessment of MOTOR POWER
   (a) Initially for groups of muscle
   (b) And then for individual muscle

Inspection

- Examine the patient while lying down, sitting, and standing and by placing the limbs in a symmetrical position.
- Evaluate for limb position, e.g., hemiplegic position (flexion in upper limb and extension in lower limb) or pseudohypertrophy (increased bulk but weaker muscle usually due to infiltration of adipose tissue in the muscle).
- Evaluate for wasting (proximal or distal, unilateral or bilateral, symmetrical, or asymmetrical).
- Bulk can also be assessed by measuring the circumference of the limbs and comparing both the limbs at equidistant points. This is conducted by checking the circumference bilaterally at fixed distances from bony points, e.g., 7 cm above the olecranon process and 10 cm below the olecranon and 15 cm above the superior edge of the patella and 10 cm below the tibial tuberosity.
- Look for fasciculations—fine subcutaneous rippling of the muscle and may be elicited by lightly tapping the muscle being observed.
- Observe for contractures (fixed deformities) and pes cavus.

Tone

Tone is the resistance to passive stretching in the muscle in a relaxed state. It is maintained by the involuntary gamma loop. Muscle spindles (intrafusal fibers) are innervated by gamma afferents, which conduct impulses to the gamma efferent neurons situated in the anterior horn cell and in turn innervate the extrafusal muscle fibers and keep them in a certain state of contraction, which determines the resting tone of the muscle.

- Request the patient to relax the limbs. Can engage the patient in a conversation or request the patient to count backward from 100 in order to achieve the relaxed state of the muscles.
- Tone has to be evaluated by passively moving each joint in various movements and assess the resistance to the passive movement. This passive movement is conducted at various velocities (slow to rapid passive movement).
- Examination of tone should be conducted across all joints starting distally from fingers and toes and then gradually proceeding proximally at all joints.

Upper Limb

- Hold the patient's hand and or arm in the examiner's right hand and evaluate resistance of the fingers and wrist to alternating flexion and extension movement at the interphalangeal, metacarpophalangeal, and wrist joints. Conduct the test at varying speeds.
- A similar movement can be conducted as pronation–supination of forearm by holding the patient's hand.
- Tone can be also assessed by passive moment in variable directions and at varying speeds for elbow flexion-extension and shoulder flexion-extension or abduction–adduction.

Lower Limbs

- Passive flexion and extension movements of the hip, knee, and ankle are performed to assess the tone.
- With the patient lying in bed with loose limbs the legs are rotated on the bed by the palm of the examiner's hands placed on the shin and resistance to the movement should be assessed.
- Keeping examiner's arm below the patient's knee in the popliteal fossa, a sudden high amplitude upward jerk is made to suddenly flex the knee upward. In normal patients, the legs are pulled back on the couch and in patients with spasticity the leg rises en bloc along with the knee with a slow fall or a "hang up." (Figs. 6.2 and 6.3)

Disorders of Tone

1. Hypotonia
   (a) Seen in LMN lesions from anterior horn cell to nerve and also in muscle disorders.
   (b) In spinal shock stage of UMN lesions.
   (c) Cerebellar lesions.
2. Increased tone

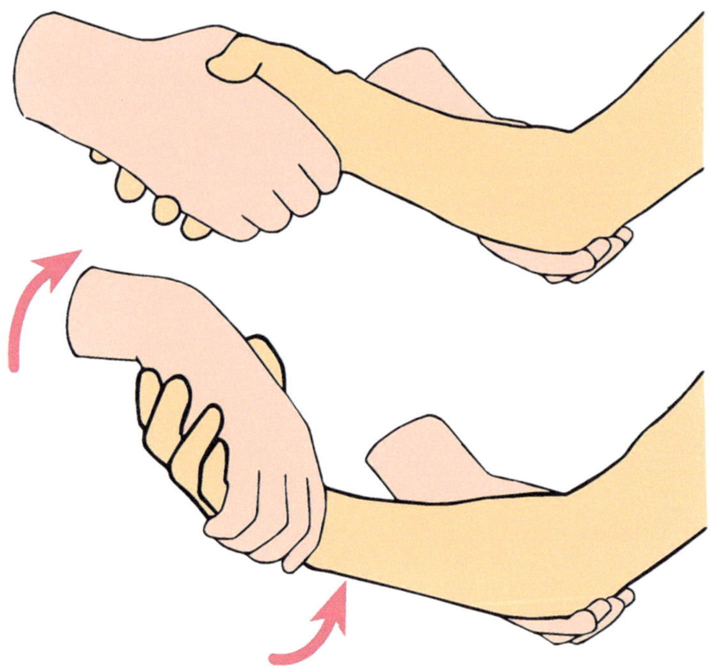

Fig. 6.2 Tone in upper limbs by rolling the wrist

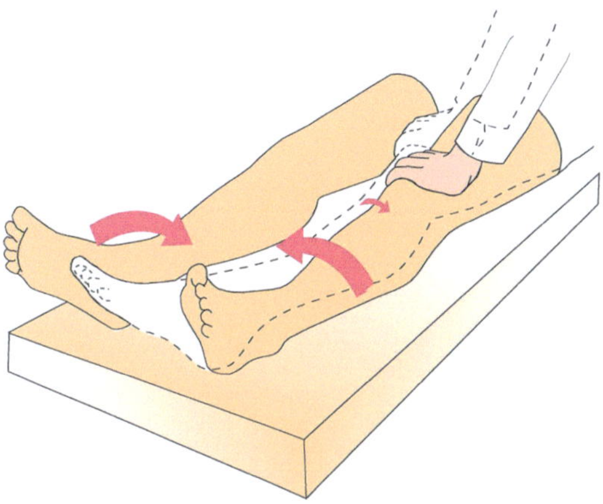

Fig. 6.3 Tone in lower limbs by rotating the limb

	Type	Lesion
Spasticity	(i) Clasp knife (resistance most when initial passive movement is made and then is suddenly overcome) (ii) Flexor muscles in upper limb and extensor muscles in lower limbs	Pyramidal lesion
Lead pipe rigidity	Hypertonia uniform throughout the movement	Extrapyramidal lesion
Cogwheel rigidly	Cogwheel rigidity of jerky nature with high or low tone due to alternate action of agonist and antagonist contraction	Extrapyramidal lesion
Myotonia	Failure of muscle contraction to relax	Muscle disorder, e.g., myotonic dystrophy
Gegenhalten	Progressive increase in resistance to passive movement proportionate to force applied by the examiner	Frontal lobe syndrome

Motor Power

- Motor power is first evaluated in *major groups* of muscles, e.g., extensors, or flexors of shoulder elbow, or knee.

NECK	• Flexion and Extension • Lateral flexion and rotation
SHOULDER	• Abduction and adduction • Rotation
ELBOW	• Flexion and extension
WRIST	• Flexion and extension • Pronation and Supination
FINGERS	• Grip • Finger flexion and extension • Abduction and adduction
ABDOMINAL MUSCLES	• Flexion and Extension of upper, middle, and lower abdominal muscles
HIP	• Flexion and Extension • Abduction and adduction
KNEE	• Flexion and Extension
ANKLE	• Dorsiflexion and plantar flexion (extension) • Eversion and Inversion
TOES	• Flexion and extension • Abduction and adduction

- *Individual muscle* testing is conducted for the group of muscles revealing the defective movement. This is of special importance in patients with motor loss due to involvement of the lower motor neuron or muscle.
- Classification of motor weakness is conducted according to the definition provided by the *Medical Research Council* (MRC).

0	Total paralysis
1	Flicker of muscle contraction but no resultant movement at the joint
2	Muscle and joint movement only with eliminated gravity
3	Normal movement against gravity but not against resistance
4	Normal movement against partial resistance
5	Normal power

6.1 Muscles of Head, Neck, and Face

These muscles of the face, neck (sternocleidomastoid and trapezius) are supplied by the cranial nerves and have been explained in the cranial nerve section.

6.2 Muscles of Upper Limb

Even though individual muscles have multiple roots supplying them, the dominant root has been indicated for purpose of evaluation.

Root	Muscles innervated by the root
C5	Rhomboids, Biceps, supraspinatus, infraspinatus deltoid
C6	Brachioradialis
C7	Triceps Long Extensors of wrist Latissimus dorsi
C8	Finger flexion
T1	Small muscles of hand

C5 dominant innervated muscles

Muscles	Segment supply/ nerve	Method
Rhomboids (Fig. 6.4)	C5 N to rhomboids	Patient places a hand on hip and pushes the elbow backward against the examiner's resistance (DIAGRAM)
Supraspinatus (Fig. 6.5)	C5 Suprascapular nerve	Initiate abduction of the arm from the side (initial 15°) against resistance (DIAGRAM)
Infraspinatus (Fig. 6.6)	C5 Suprascapular nerve	Flex the elbow and dig it into the trunk and hold the elbow in contact with the trunk. Externally rotate the forearm outward against resistance (DIAGRAM)
Deltoid (Fig. 6.7)	C5 Circumflex nerve	Hold the arm abducted to >45° and raise against resistance (DIAGRAM)
Biceps (Fig. 6.8)	C5 Musculocutaneous nerve	Flex the elbow against resistance (DIAGRAM)

Muscles	Innervation segment supply/nerve	Method
C6 Dominant innervated muscles		
Brachioradialis (Fig. 6.9)	C6 (C5) Radial nerve	Pronate the hand to bring the thumb toward the nose against resistance (diagram)
Serratus anterior (Fig. 6.10)	C6 (C5, C7) N to Serratus anterior	The patient pushes the wall with both arms forward against resistance. Observe for serratus anterior contraction/ winging
C7 Dominant innervated		
Muscles		
Triceps (Fig. 6.11)	C7 (C6, C8) Radial N	Extend the elbow against resistance
Lattismus dorsi	C7 N to Lattismus dorsi	Abduct the arm to 90° and patient abducts it against resistance
Long finger extensors		
Extensor digitorum	C7 (C8) Radial	Extend the fingers at metacarpo phalangeal joint against resistance
Extensor carpi ulnaris	C7 (C8) Radial	Hold the fingers extended with dorsiflexion of wrist toward radial side
Extension carpi radialis longus	C7 (C8) Radial	Fingers extended with dorsiflexion of wrist to upper side (Figs. 6.12, 6.13 and 6.14)
C8 Dominant innervated muscles		
Long finger flexors		
Flexor digitorum superticialis Flexor digitorum profundus	C8 Median and ulnar N	Flexion of fingers at metacarpophalangeal joint and wrist
Flexor carpi ulnaris	C8 Ulnar	Flexion of metacarpophalangeal joint of mesial finger
Flexor carpi radialis	C7 C8 Median	Flexion of fingers and wrist toward radial side (Figs. 6.15, 6.16, 6.17 and 6.18)

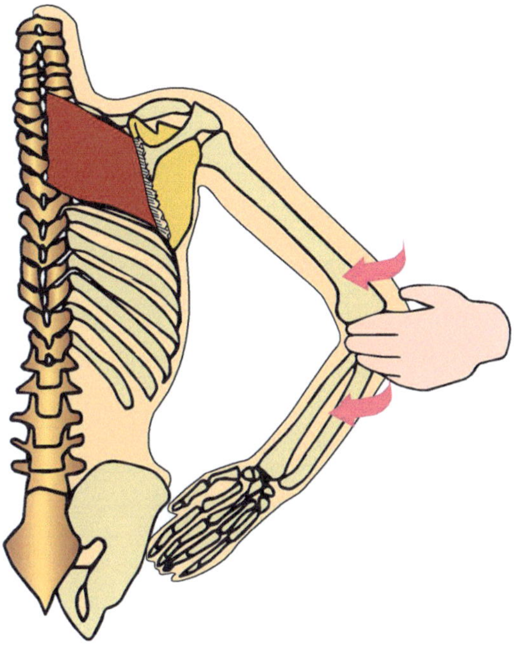

Fig. 6.4 Rhomboids: pull elbow backwards

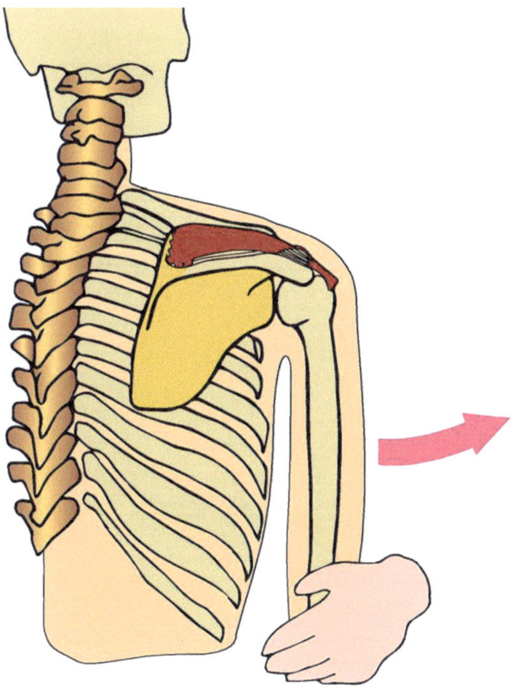

Fig. 6.5 Supraspinatus: initial 15 degree abduction of arm

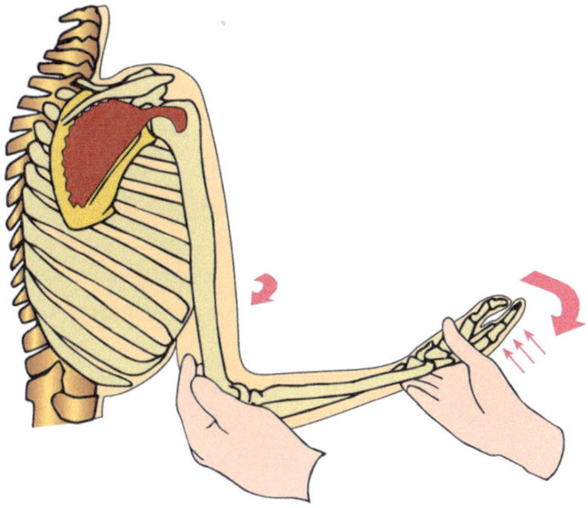

Fig. 6.6 Infraspinatus: dig elbow into the trunk and externally rotate the forearm

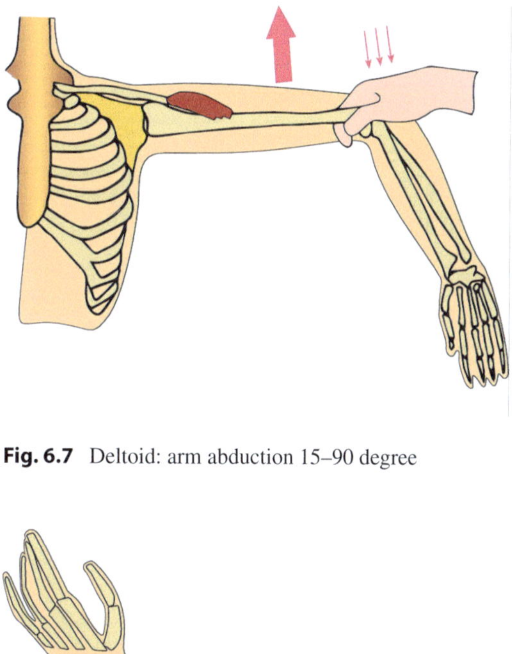

Fig. 6.7 Deltoid: arm abduction 15–90 degree

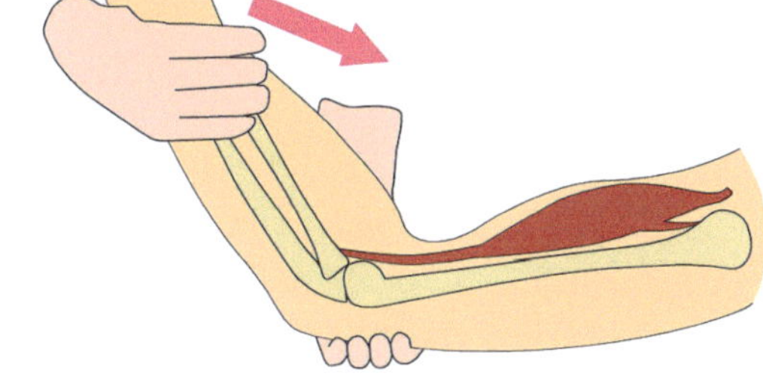

Fig. 6.8 Biceps- flexion at elbow

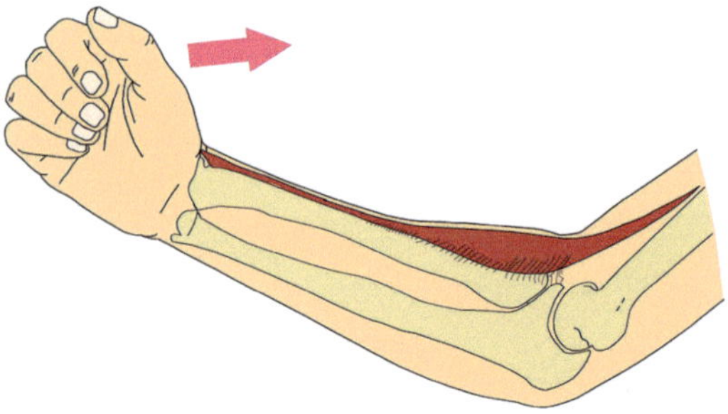

Fig. 6.9 Brachioradialis: flex elbow in semipronation: thumb to nose

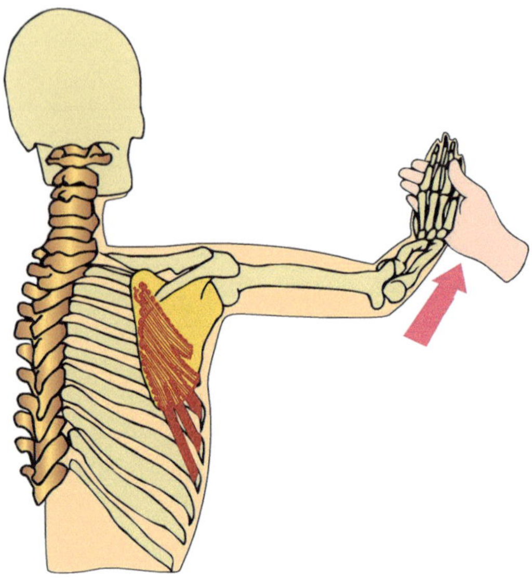

Fig. 6.10 Serratus anterior: push forward with extended elbow

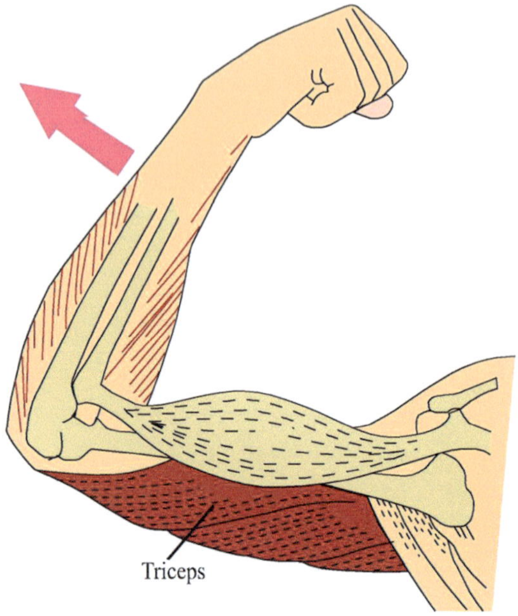

Fig. 6.11 triceps extension at elbow

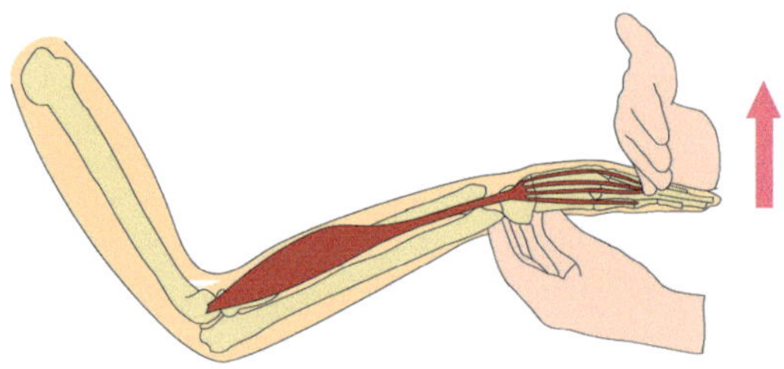

Fig. 6.12 Evaluating finger extensors

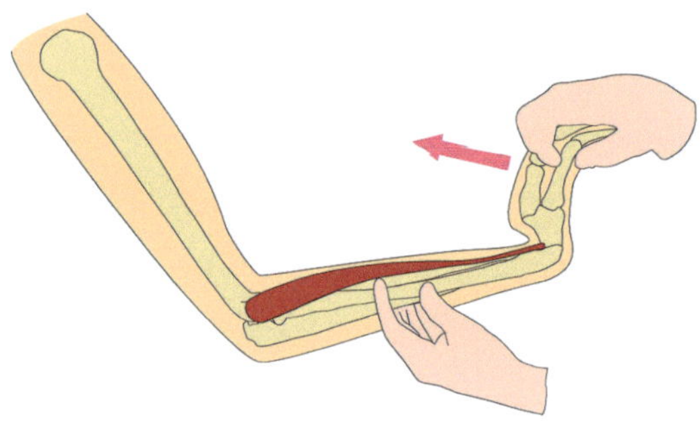

Fig. 6.13 Evaluating wrist extension

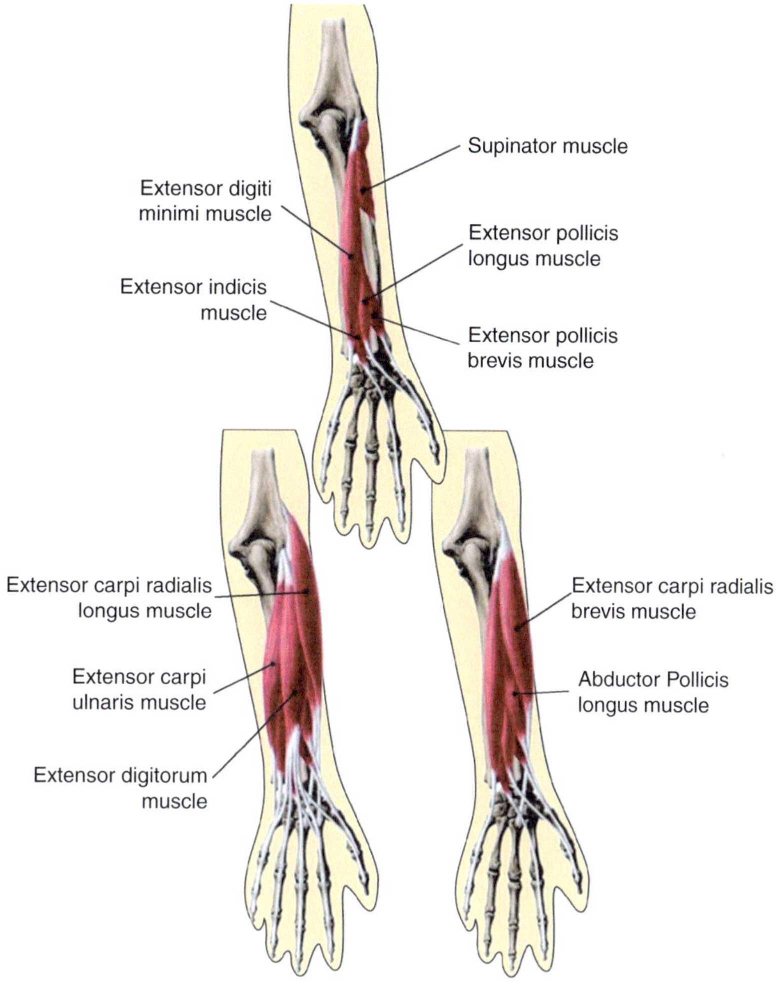

Fig. 6.14 Extensor muscle of forearm

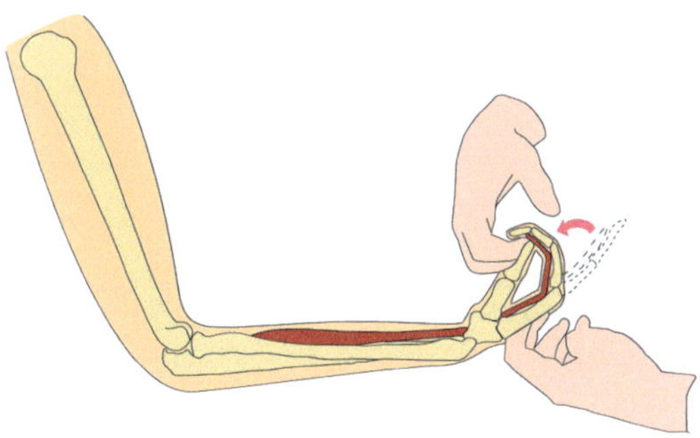

Fig. 6.15 Evaluating finger flexors

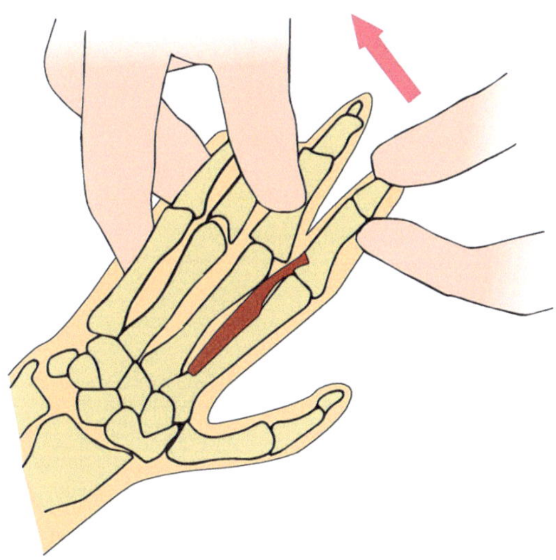

Fig. 6.16 Evaluating finger adduction

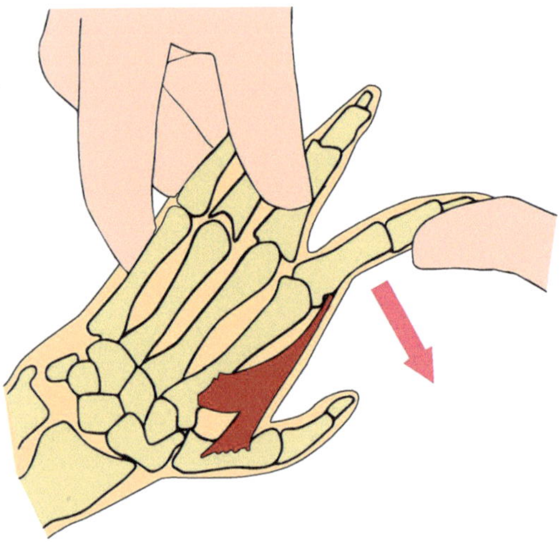

Fig. 6.17 Evaluating finger adduction

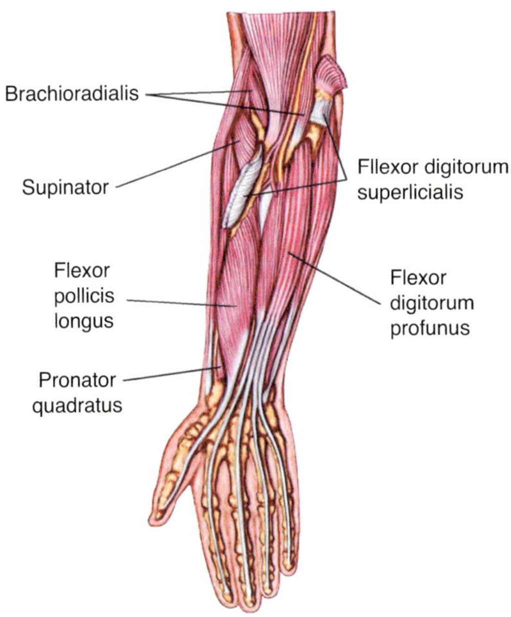

Fig. 6.18 Flexor muscles of forearm

T1 Dominant Muscles

Muscles	Segment supply/nerve	Method
Muscles of thumb	Median nerve innervated "LOAF" Ulnar N– Radial N–	Lateral 2 lumbricals, opponens pollicis, abductor pollicis brevis, flexor pollicis longus
Opponens policis	T1 Median N	Press little fingertip and thumb to make a ring

Muscles	Segment supply/nerve	Method
Abductor pollicis brevis	T1 Median N	• Place an object between thumb and index finger to prevent full adduction • Attempt to raise the thumb upward against resistance
Flexor pollicis longus	C5 Median	Flex the distal phallanx of the thumb against resistance
Lumbricals (Lateral 2)	C8 T1 Median N	Flex the extended finger at meta-carpophalangeal joints
Radial nerve		
Extensor pollicis longus	C8 Radial N	Extend the thumb at meta-carpophalangeal joint
Abductor policis longus	C8 Radial N	Abduct the thumb against resistance
Ulnar Nerve		
Mesial lumbricals	C8 T1 Ulnar N	Flex the extended fingers at meta-carpophalangeal joint
Interosceii	C 8 T1 Ulnar N	Abducting fingers
Abductor policis	T1 ulnar	Hold firmly a paper between thumb and palm
Abductor digiti minimi	T1 ulnar	Place hand palm upward on table and abduct the little finger (Figs. 6.19, 6.20 and 6.21)

6.3 Muscles of Trunk

1. *Abdominal muscles*—nerve supply D5–D12 root

    Patient attempts to raise the head and chest while lying down and the examiner inspects and palpates the contraction of the upper abdominal muscles.

    Next, while lying down the patient raises together both legs above the bed and the examiner inspects and palpates the contraction of the lower abdominal muscles.

2. *Extensors of the spine*—Nerve supply D1–D12

    Patient lies prone and raises the shoulder and upper chest above the bed and extensor

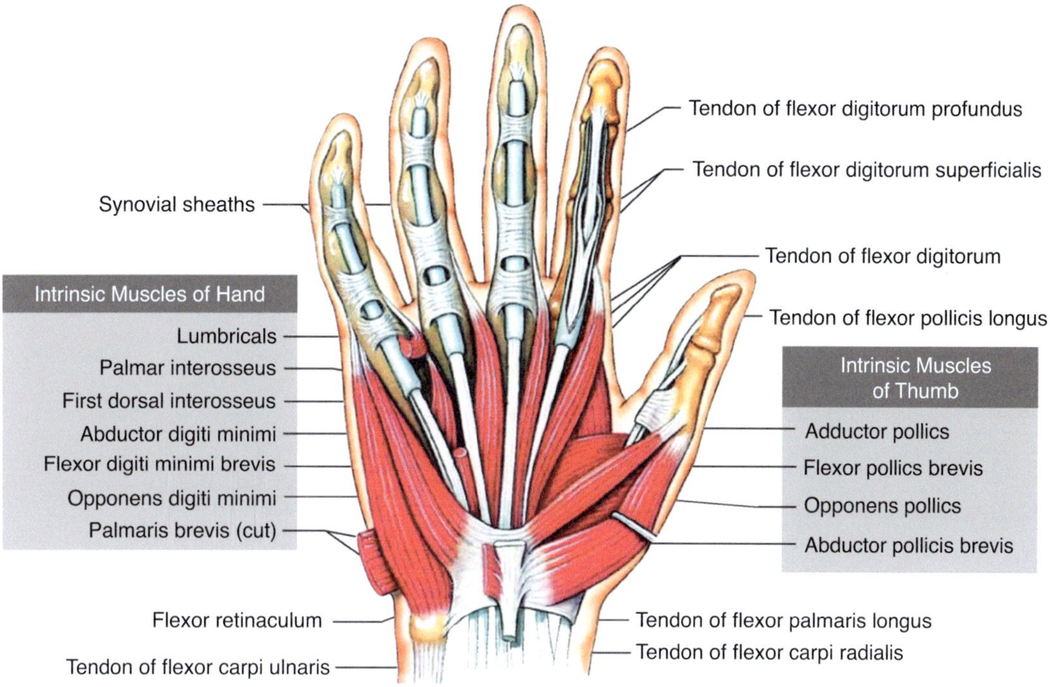

Fig. 6.19 Intrinsic muscles of hand

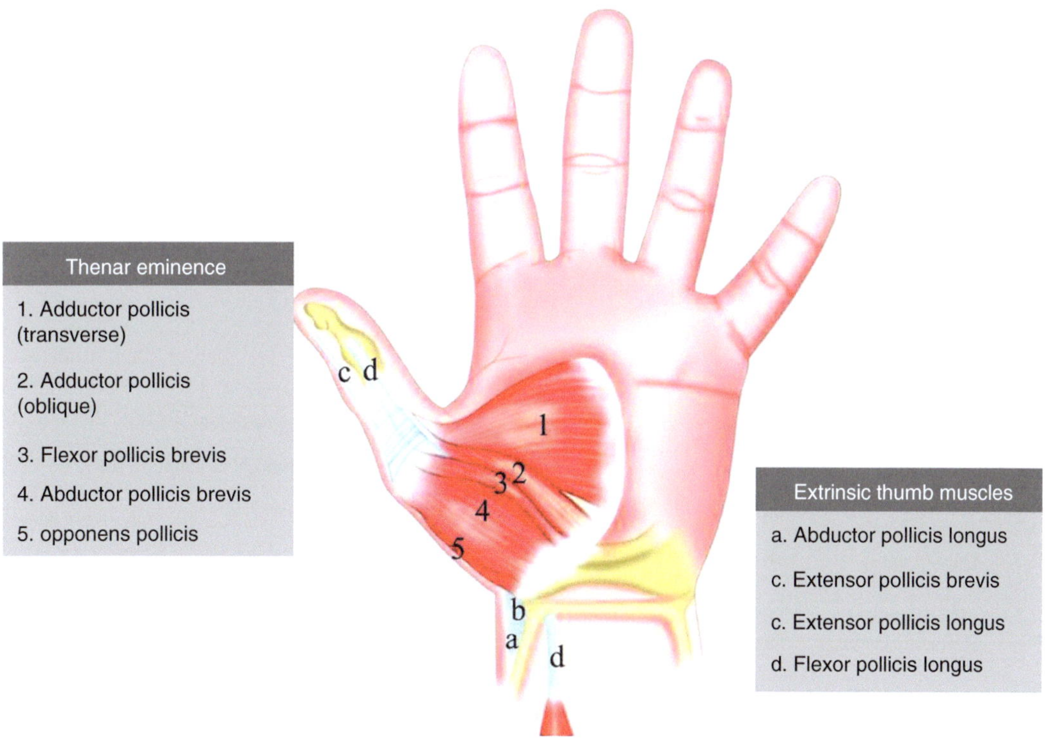

Fig. 6.20 Extrinsic and intrinsic muscles of thumb

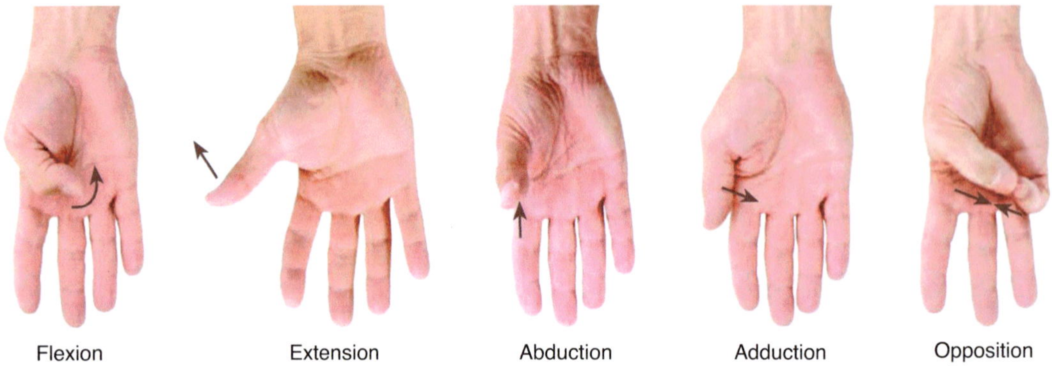

Fig. 6.21 Movements of the thumb

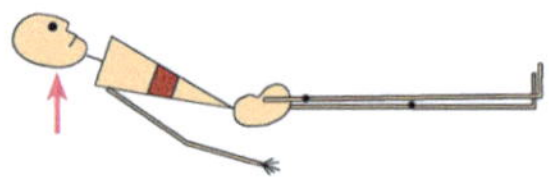

Fig. 6.22 Evaluating upper abdominal muscle strength

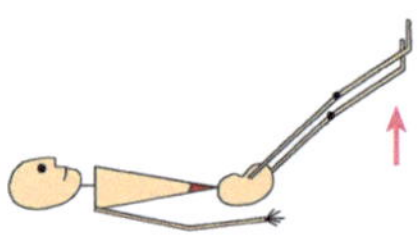

Fig. 6.23 Evaluating lower abdominal muscle strength

muscles of the upper back are inspected and palpated. Next the patient then raises both legs above the bed and again extensor muscles of lower back are inspected and palpated.

3. *Intercostal muscles* nerve supply D1–D12

   Observe the movement of the chest on quiet and deep inspiration and expiration (Figs. 6.22 and 6.23).

6.4 Muscles of Lower Limb

L1 L2	Iliacus, psoas major, rectus femoris	Hip flexion
L3 L4	Quadriceps	Knee extension
L5	EHL (Extensor Hallucis Longus)	• Dorsiflexion of foot • Inversion, eversion of ankle • Extension of big toe
S1		Hip extension knee flexion planter flexion

Muscles	Innervation segment supply/nerve	Method
Hip flexion iliopsoas (Fig. 6.24)	L1,2 Lumbosacral plexus	• Lift the knee toward the chest and maintain the knee at 90° • Pull the thigh against resistance
Hip extension—gluteus maximus (Fig. 6.25)	L5 S1 Interior gluteal N	Lying supine with straight legs, patient pushes the leg into the bed against the resistance of the examiner's hand
Hip abduction—gluteus medius and minimus (Fig. 6.26)	L4 L5 Superior gluteal N	Take the leg outward at the hip with resistance by the examiner on the ankle and fixing the opposite ankle
Hip adduction—adductor magnus (Fig. 6.27)	L2 L3 Obturator N	Patient keeps both ankles together. One ankle is fixed and keeps the other ankle approximated while the examiner tries to pull it out
Knee extension—quadriceps femoris (Fig. 6.28)	L3, 4 Femoral N	Flex the knee to 90° support the knee with one hand and place the other on the patient's ankle and ask the patient to straighten the leg, at the knee against resistance
Knee flexion—hamstrings (Fig. 6.29)	L5 S1 Sciatic nerve	Patient bends the knee and bring the heel toward the hip against resistance

Muscles	Innervation segment supply/nerve	Method
Foot dorsiflexion—tibialis another (Fig. 6.30)	L 5 (L4) Deep peroneal N	Patient pulls the ankle and toes toward his/her head against resistance
Foot plantar flexion—gastrocnemius (Fig. 6.31)	S 1 Posterior tibial N	Patient pushes toes and foot downward against resistance
Foot eversion—peroneus longus and brevis (Fig. 6.32)	L 5 S1 Superficial peroneal N	Patient turns the foot outward
Foot inversion (Fig. 6.33)	L4 L5 Posterior tibial N	Patient turns the foot inwards
Big toe extension Extensor hallucis longus (Fig. 6.34)	L5 Deep peroneal N	Patient pulls the big toe toward his/her head against resistance
Extension of toes Extensor digtorum brevis (Figs. 6.35, 6.36, 6.37 and 6.38)	L5 S1 Deep peroneal N	Patient pulls all toes toward his/her head against resistance

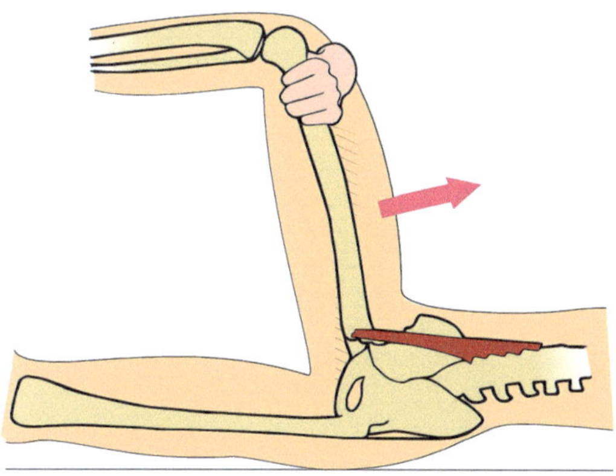

Fig. 6.24 Evaluating hip flexors

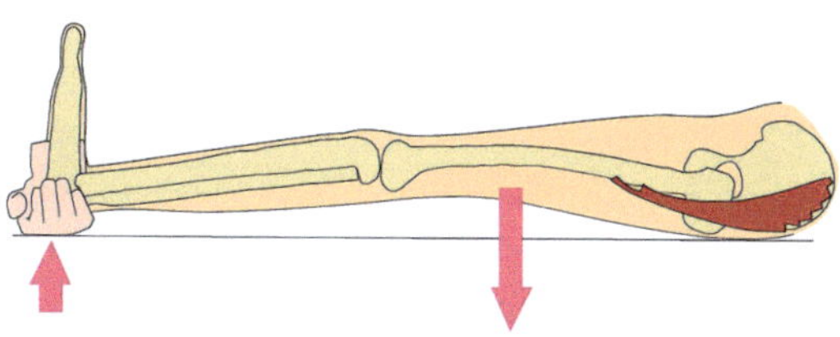

Fig. 6.25 Evaluating hip extensors

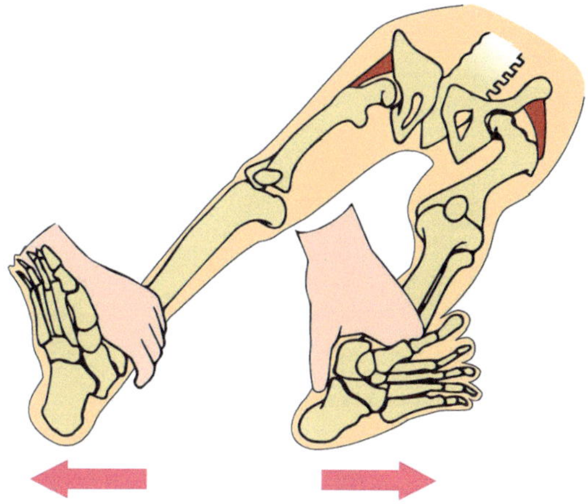

Fig. 6.26 Evaluating hip abductors

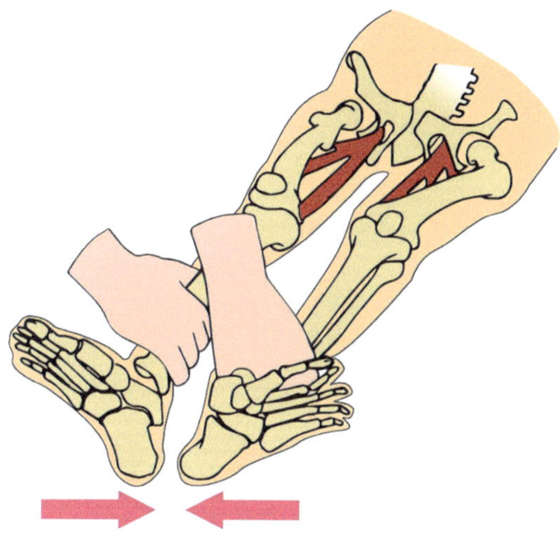

Fig. 6.27 Evaluating hip adductors

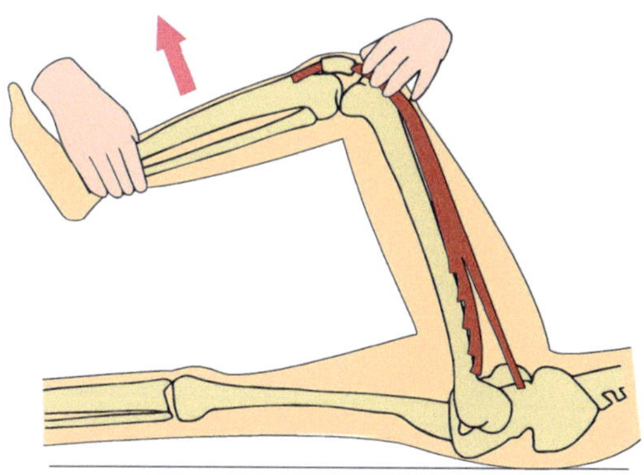

Fig. 6.28 Evaluating knee extensors

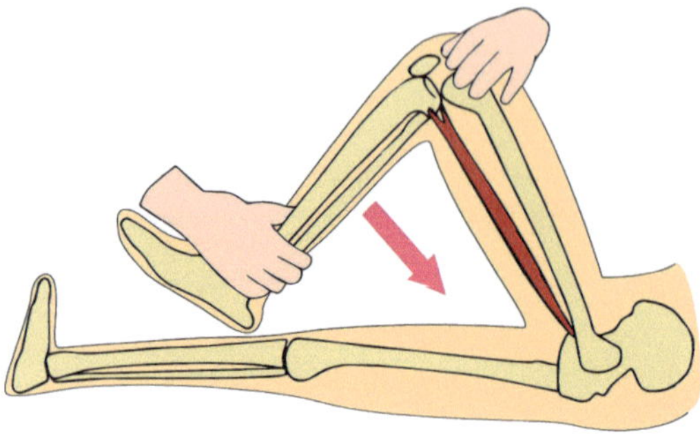

Fig. 6.29 Evaluating knee flexors

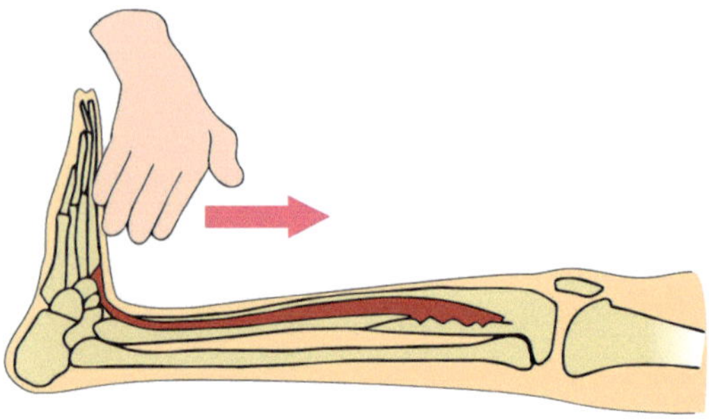

Fig. 6.30 Evaluating dorsiflexion of foot

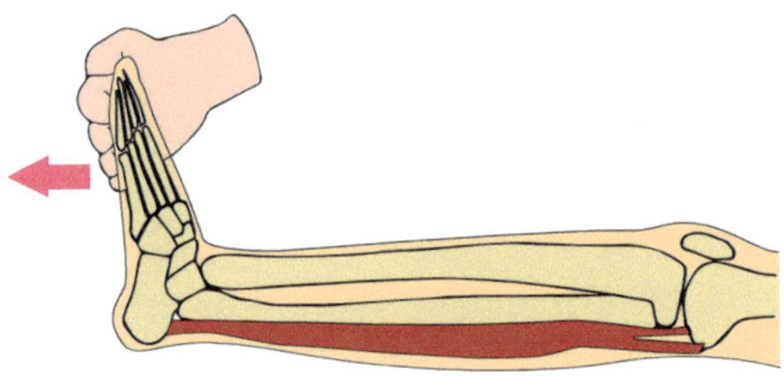

Fig. 6.31 Evaluating plantar flexion of foot

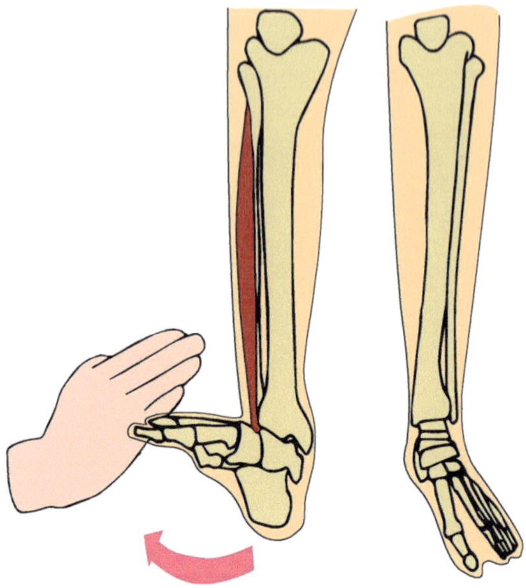

Fig. 6.32 Evaluating eversion of foot

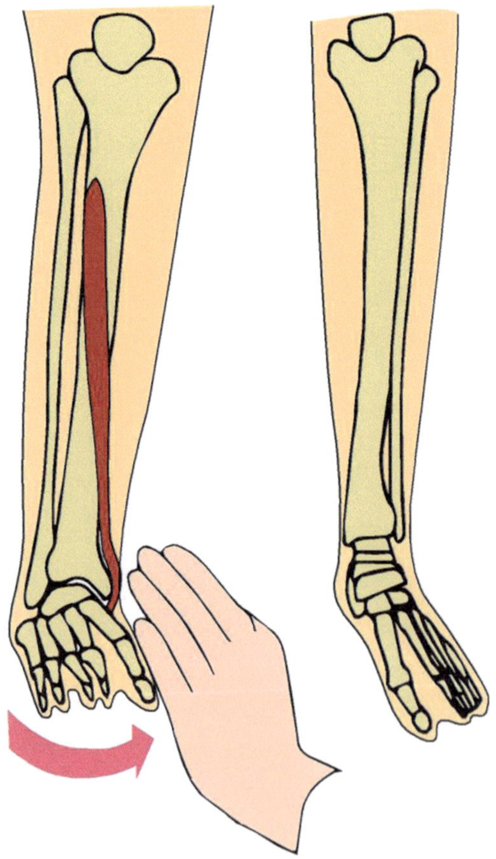

Fig. 6.33 Evaluating inversion of foot

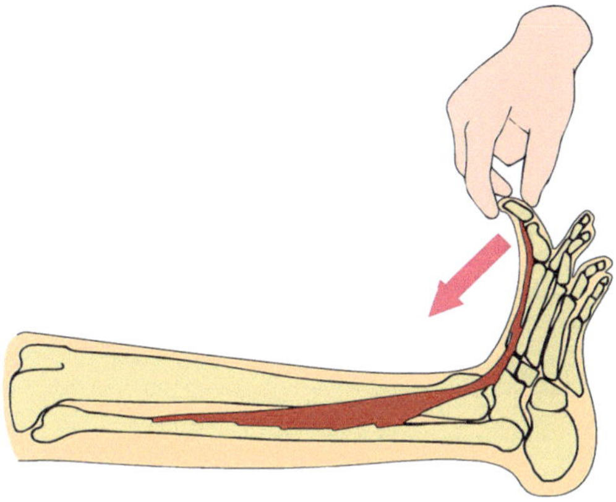

Fig. 6.34 Evaluating extensor of big toe (EHL)

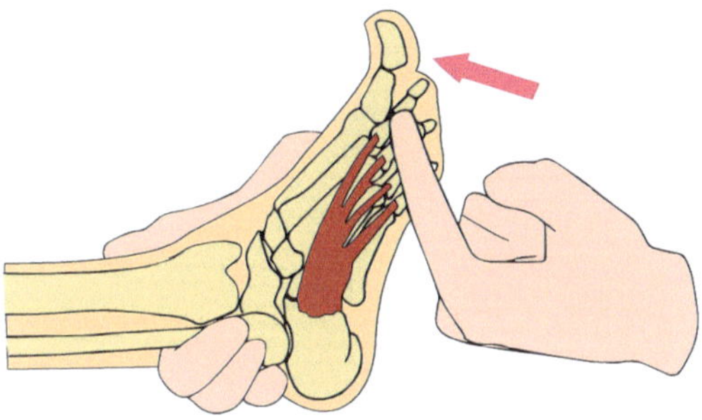

Fig. 6.35 Evaluating extensors of toes

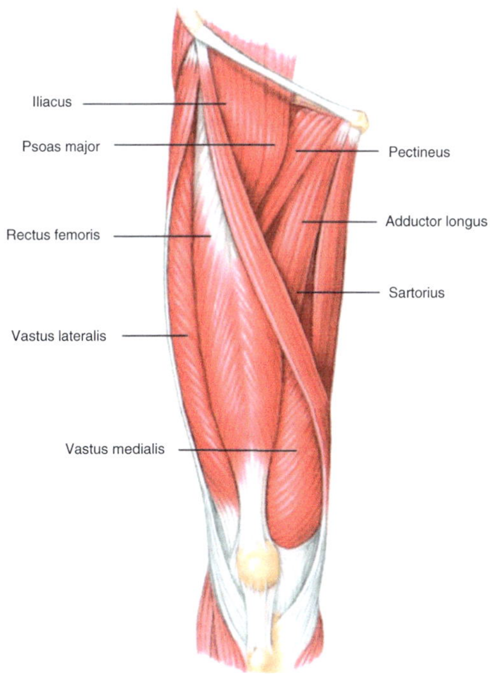

Fig. 6.36 Muscles of anterior thigh

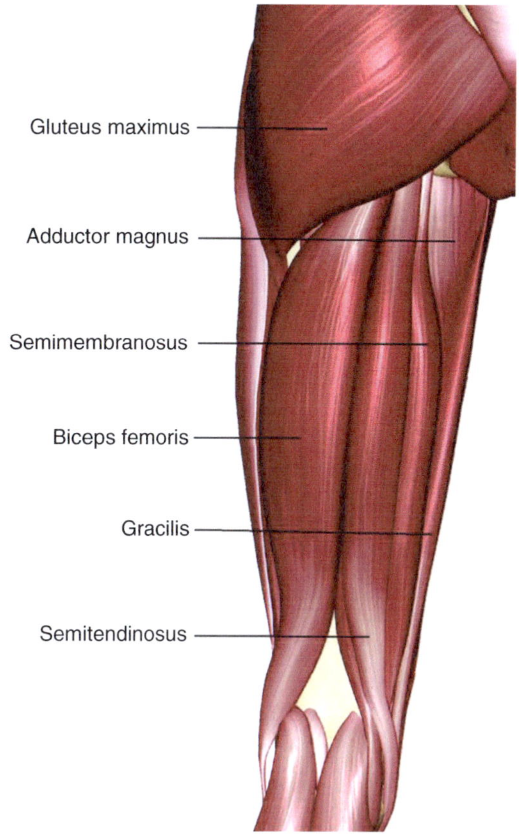

Fig. 6.37 Muscles of posterior thigh

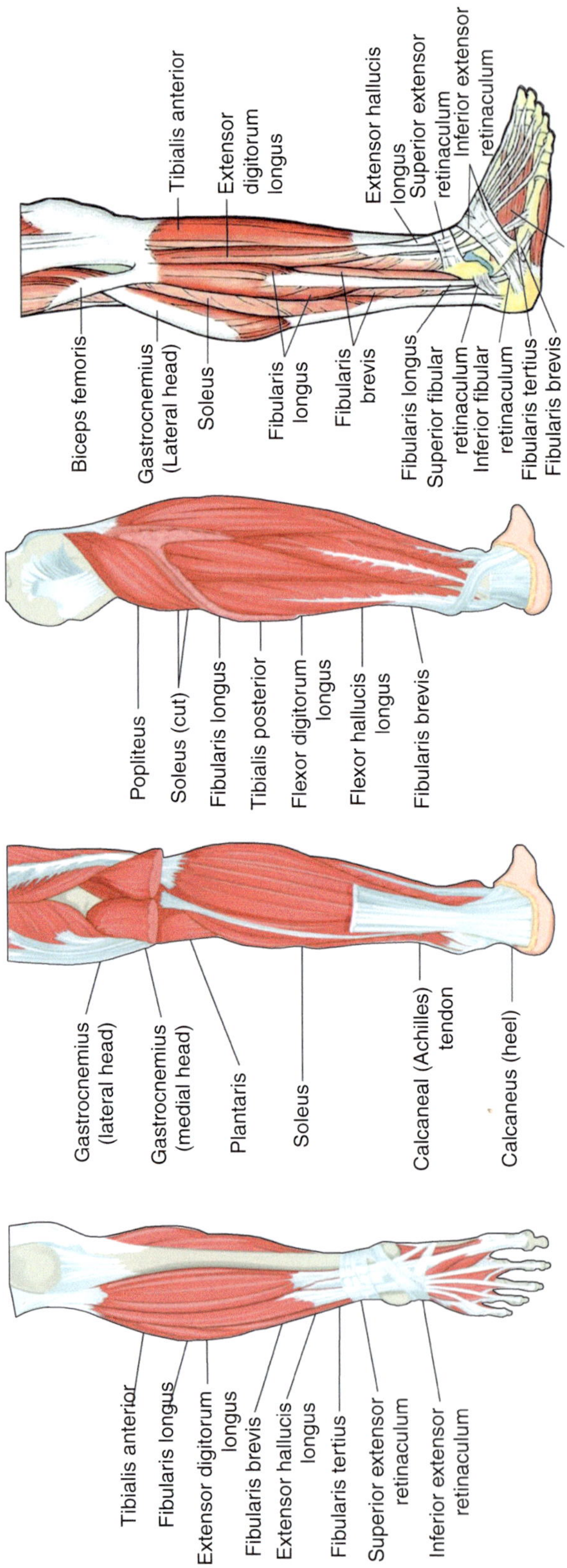

Fig. 6.38 Muscles of leg

7 Reflexes

The major purpose of the examination of superficial and deep tendon reflexes is to distinguish between central nervous system disorders from peripheral nervous system disorders (UMN lesion from LMN).

Reflexes require a stimulus, an afferent pathway, a link with the motor (efferent) pathway, a motor neuron, and a contractile or other effector elements. Most reflexes are influenced by higher centers. Pattern of abnormality of the reflexes can help in localizing the site of breach. This breach may be in the local reflex arc or due to an abnormal input from the higher centers.

7.1 Superficial Reflexes

These are *polysynaptic* reflexes involving the CNS and are elicited by stimulation of the skin or mucous membrane and result in contraction of one or more muscles. They are polysynaptic reflexes and are lost in lesions of the corticospinal tract or when the local sensory or motor arc is disrupted. They are not dependent on the stimulation of tendons or muscles (Fig. 7.1).

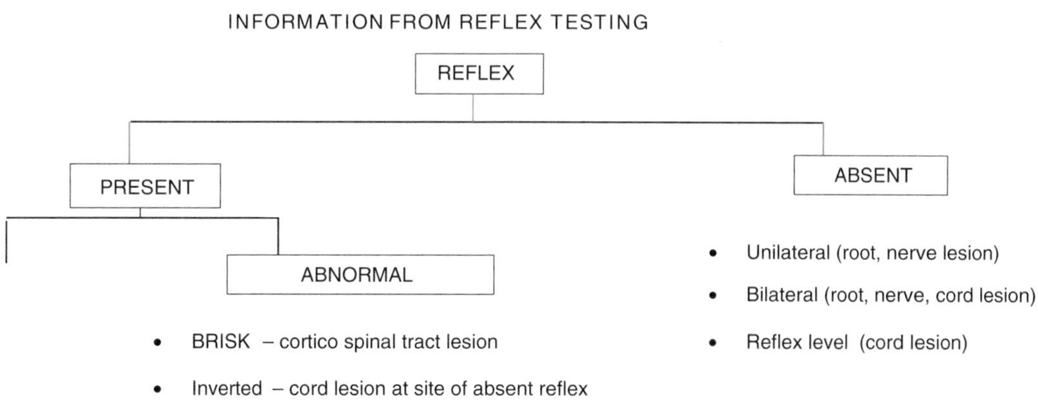

V. Suri, *Clinical Neurological Examination and Localization*,
https://doi.org/10.1007/978-981-16-1228-2_7

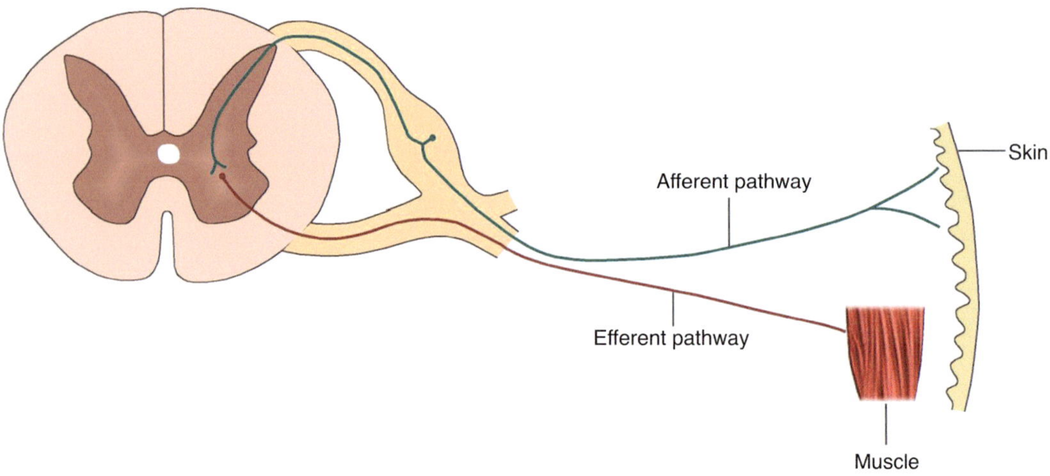

Fig. 7.1 Superficial reflex (stimulation of skin with contraction of muscle-polysynaptic pathway

Reflex	Afferent	Efferent
Corneal	5th cranial N	7th cranial N
Conjunctival	5th cranial N	7th cranial N
Pharyngeal or gag	9th cranial N	10th cranial N
Abdominal reflex	Epigastric T7–9 roots Upper abdominal T9–11 Lower abdominal D11–D12	T7–9 roots T9–11 roots D11–L1 roots
Cremasteric (L1, 2)	Femoral nerve	Pudendal nerve
Bulbocavernosus (S3/4) (squeezing the tip of glans penis leads to contraction of bulbocavernosus muscle)	Pudendal N	Pudendal N
Anal reflex S4, S5 (stroking perianal skin causes contraction of external anal sphincter)	Pudental N	Pudental N
Plantar reflex L5 S1	Posterior tibial N	Posterior tibial N

7.1.1 Abdominal Reflex (T1–T12)

- Patient should lie flat with flexed knees and is asked to relax the abdomen, which is ascertained by palpation. Patient is explained the procedure.
- Stroke the abdomen gently by stimulating *only the skin* and not the underlying muscle from outer quadrant to medial aspect in upper, middle, and lower abdomen by using a blunt object, e.g., tongue depressor, orange stick, or two point discrimination.

  Normal result–Contraction of underlying muscle and pulling of the umbilicus toward the stimulation.

  Abnormal response–Absent in
  - Pyramidal lesion
  - Local reflex arc root lesion

Segmental innervation
- Epigastric T7–9 roots
- Upper abdominal T9–11
- Lower abdominal T11–12 (Fig. 7.2)

7.1.2 Cremasteric Reflex (L1)

- Upper and inner thigh is stroked in a downward and inward direction with a blunt orange stick, back of a hammer, or two point discriminator.
- *Normal result*–Contraction of cremasteric muscle pulling up the ipsilateral scrotum and testicle.
- Segment innovation L1
- *Abnormal response*–Absent in pyramidal lesion above L1 or local L1 root pathology.

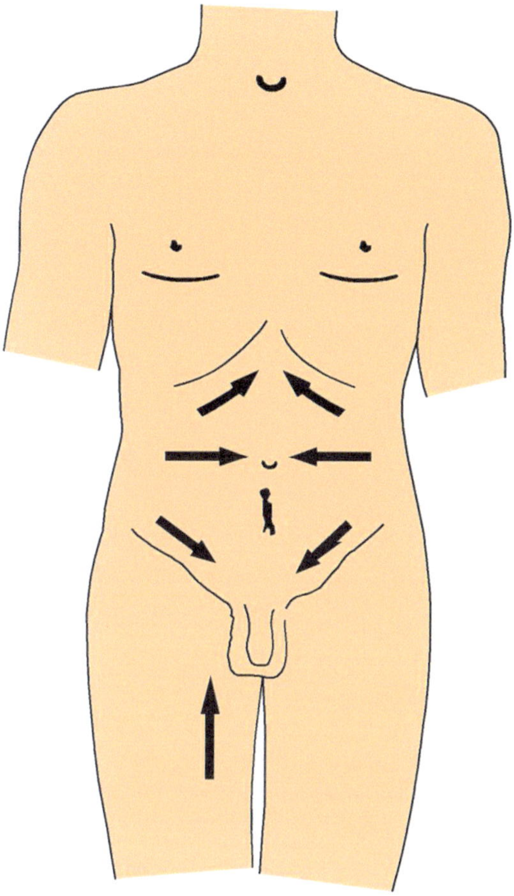

Fig. 7.2 Superficial reflexes (abdominal and cremasteric reflexes)

7.1.3 Anal Reflex (S4/5)

- Lightly stroke the perianal skin.
- *Normal result*–contraction of the external anal sphincter Segment innervation-S4-5.
- *Abnormal*–absent in pyramidal lesion above S4/5 or local arc pathology.

7.1.4 Bulbocavernosus (S3/4)

- Squeeze the glans penis
- Normal result—contraction of the bulbocavernosus muscle.
- Abnormal—absent contraction

7.1.5 Plantar Response or Babinski Response (S1)

This is the most important reflex to be elicited since it is the prototypical finding of corticospinal tract disease.

- Patient is made to lie down with slight flexion of the knees and external rotation of the leg so that the outer aspect of the foot touches the bed.
- Explain to the patient that the sole will be stimulated and that attempt should be made by the patient to relax the foot.
- A blunt object, e.g., orange stick, back of percussion hammer, or two point discriminator is used to firmly and briskly stroke the lateral aspect of the sole starting from the heel area and moving up to the ball of the toes and stopping short of the base of the big toe. The movement of the big toe, other toes, and tensor fascia lata in the thigh is observed.

Segment innervation S1 (L5) (Figs. 7.3 and 7.4)

Normal response (Flexor Plantar response)

- Big toe will flex at the meta tarso phalangeal joint.
- Other toes will also flex and close together.
- Response should not start immediately at the start of the stimulation (which would indicate a likely Withdrawal response).

Abnormal response (Extensor Plantar or positive Babinski response)

1. *No response*
   (a) Thick sole.
   (b) Absent sensation on sole.
   (c) Severe LMN motor weakness of foot muscles resulting in complete weakness of extensor muscles of the foot.
   (d) Bony deformities in the foot, e.g., surgically corrected hallux valgus or bony ankylosis of toes (observe movement of

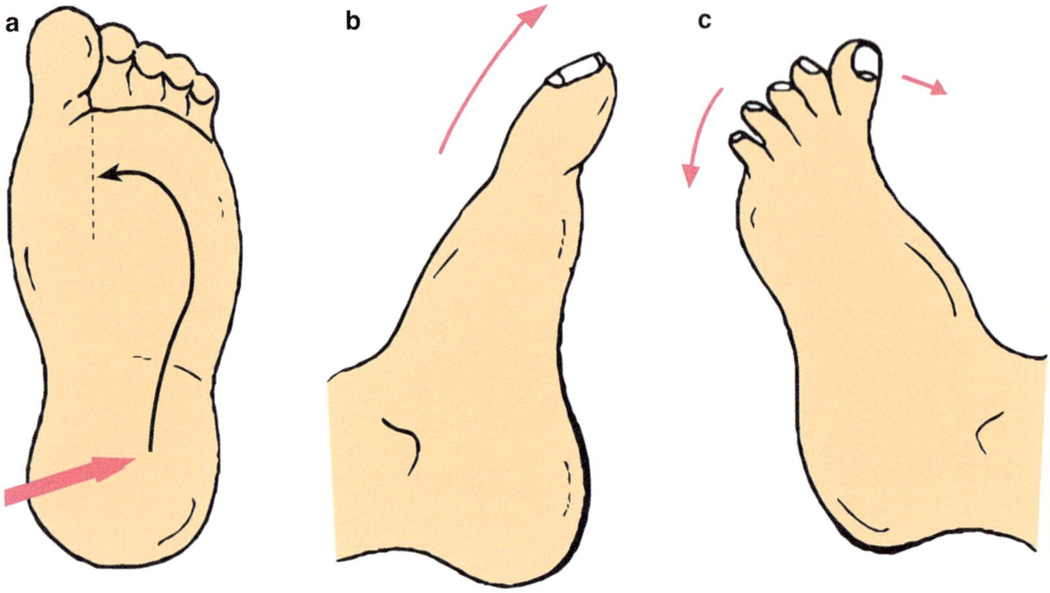

Fig. 7.3 Plantar reflex (**a**), (**b**), (**c**)

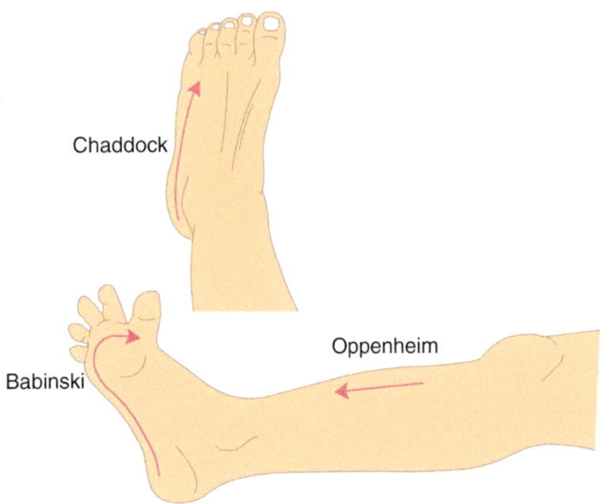

Fig. 7.4 Alternative plantar reflexes

other toes and other muscles, e.g., tensor facia lata).

2. *Withdrawal reflex* immediate initiation of reflex as soon as the sole is touched with extension of big toe, ankle dorsiflexion and leg flexion, and en bloc flexion of the leg.
3. *Extensor response or positive Babinski response*
   (a) Extension of the big toe at metatarsophalangeal joint
   (b) Fanning and dorsiflexion of other toes
   (c) Visible or palpable contraction of tensor fascia lata in the thigh

Clinical Value

- Indicates a corticospinal tract (UMN) lesion from brain to L5 segment of cord.
- Maybe seen normally in infants below the age of 6 months.

Segmental Innervation

- Afferent: Sensory stimulus in S1 dermatome travelling up in Posterior tibial nerve to Sciatic N and to L5S1 roots and synapse in anterior horn cell to elicit the motor response.

Efferent: Motor root L5S1 from anterior horn to Sciatic nerve to Posterior tibial N (toe flexors), deep peroneal N (Extensor hallucis longus, Extensor digitorum longus).

Plantar reflex can be elicited by several other methods with similar inference.

- Chaddock sign—stroking the lateral malleolus.
- Gordon sign—squeezing the calf muscle
- Oppenheim sign—applying downward moving pressure on tibia (medial more than lateral).
- Throckmorten reflex—percussion over the metatarsophalangeal joint of the big toe.

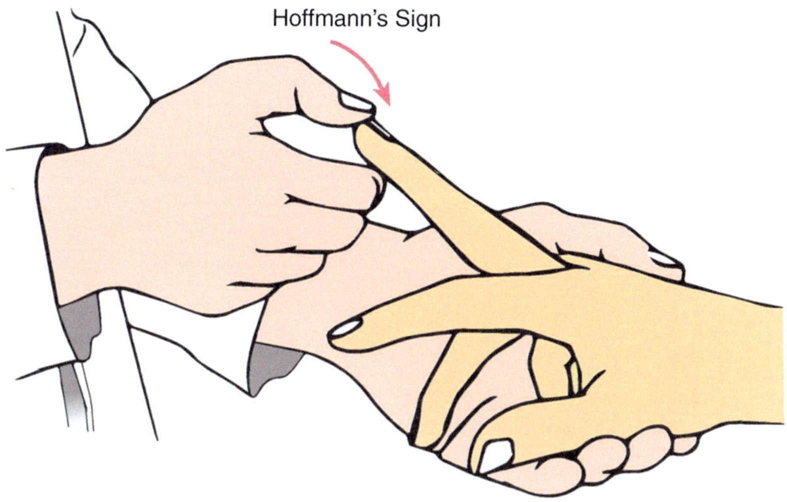

Fig. 7.5 Hoffman reflex

The Hoffman Reflex

Elicited by flicking down the terminal phalanx of the patient's middle finger between the examiner's thumb and index finger is described as the upper limb equivalent of the plantar response by a number of neurologists.

It is important to mention that the Hoffman reflex is considered as a monosynaptic spinal reflex (deep tendon reflex) involving the Flexor digitorum profundus muscle by some neurologists and is not considered equivalent to the polysynaptic plantar response. However, other neurologists still consider the Hoffman reflex as the upper limb equivalent of the plantar response indicative of a corticospinal tract lesion above the C5-6 level (Fig. 7.5).

7.2 Deep Tendon Reflexes

Deep tendon reflexes are *monosynaptic* stretch reflexes initiated by sudden stretching of a muscle sending impulses from the muscle spindle afferents (intrafusal fibers), which synapse directly with the motor neurons leading to contraction of the extrafusal muscle.

	Superficial reflexes	Deep tendon reflexes
Type	Polysynaptic	Monosynaptic
Stimulation	• Skin • Mucous membrane	Muscle spindle (intrafusal fibers)

	Superficial reflexes	Deep tendon reflexes
Type	Polysynaptic	Monosynaptic
UMN lesion	Absent	Brisk
LMN lesion of area	Absent	Absent

Muscle spindles are sensory end organs located within a capsule within striated muscles. They are also called *intrafusal fibers* to separate them from the usual straight muscle contractile fibers called *extrafusal fibers*. The primary and secondary sensory fibers carry impulses from the intrafusal fibers and synapse with the motor neurons in the anterior horn cell. The motor fibers innervating the extrafusal fibers are called alpha motor neurons and those innervating the spindles (intrafusal fibers) are called gamma motor neurons.

When the skeletal muscle is stretched, the intrafusal fibers of the muscle spindle are elongated and they produce an afferent sensory input that reaches the spinal cord and synapses with the Alpha motor neurons in the anterior horn cell and these cause rapid contraction of the extrafusal fibers of the stretched muscle (Fig. 7.6).

7.2.1 Reinforcement of Reflex

In the event of sluggish or absent reflex, reinforcement (by increasing the gamma motor neu-

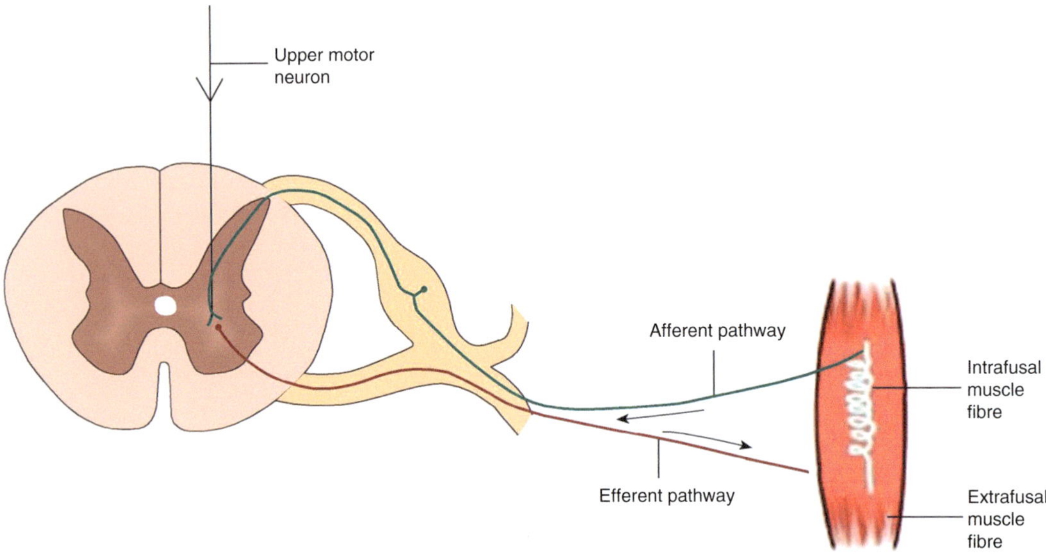

Fig. 7.6 Pathway for muscle stretch reflex on deep tendon jerk

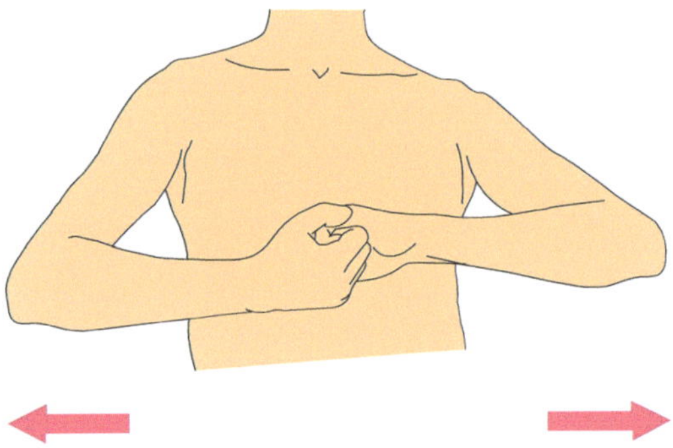

Fig. 7.7 Reinforcemnet of deep tendon reflexes

ron input to the spindles) maneuvers may elicit an absent-looking reflex.

- For arm reflexes—clenching jaws or opposite fist.
- For leg reflexes—Jendrassik maneuver-interlocking both hands and fingers and pulling them apart or clenching the teeth (Fig. 7.7).

7.2.2 Grading of Deep Tendon Reflex

- 0 = Absent despite reinforcement
- 1 = Diminished-present only with reinforcement
- 2 = Normal
- 3 = Increased (brisk)
- 4 = Markedly brisk with clonus

7.2.3 Components of a Brisk Reflex

A brisk reflex has certain components and just an increase of amplitude of the reflex alone does not necessarily signify a brisk reflex.

(a) Elicitation with a subthreshold stimulation, e.g., tapping with finger rather than hammer.
(b) Increased area of response, e.g., elbow flexion and finger flexion in biceps jerk.
(c) Increased area of stimulus—elicitation of reflex even by stimulating muscle belly (not only tendon).
(d) Increased amplitude of muscle contraction.
(e) Elicitation of Clonus

7.2.4 Inverted Reflex

The reflex is labeled as inverted when a combination of loss of reflex being tested (due to LMN lesion at that level of the cord) is accompanied with a brisk elicitation of the reflex at an immediate lower level due to hyperreflexia below the cord lesion resulting in increase in reflexogenic zone of other reflexes. It is a characteristic sign to indicate the site of lesion in the cord which is at the level of the absent reflex.

- *Inverted biceps reflex*
  - Elicitation of the Bicep reflex results in absence of elbow flexion but results in extension of the elbow due to brisk triceps reflex (indicates cord lesion at C5).
- *Inverted supinator reflex*
  - Elicitation of supinator reflex does not result in flexion of the elbow but causes finger flexion (indicates cord lesion at C6).

7.2.5 Hung Up Reflex

When the reflex elicited is slow, diminished but characteristically prolonged, it is labelled as a hung-up reflex. It is an abnormal response and is seen in hypothyroidism.

7.2.6 Pendular Jerk

Is usually used to describe increased oscillations when the knee jerk is elicited with the legs dangling above the floor. More than two and a half oscillations of the leg on eliciting the knee jerk is labelled as a pendular jerk and is seen in cerebellar lesions.

Nerves and nerve roots innervating the muscles involved in the Reflex.

	Nerve	Nerve root	Muscle
Biceps	Musculo-cutaneous	*C5* (6)	Biceps
Brachiora-dialis	Radial	*C6* (5)	Brachioradialis
Triceps	Radial	*C7* (6)	Triceps
Finger flexion	Median, Ulnar	*C8*	Finger flexors (FDS, FDP)
Knee	Femoral	*L3* (4)	Quadriceps
Ankle	Tibial N	*S1*	Gastrocnemius

1. *Biceps jerk (C5/*C6, through musculocutaneous N)
   (a) Place the arm loosely flexed on the abdomen.
   (b) Place the examiner's finger on the biceps tendon and hit your finger gently but briskly with the percussion hammer using wrist movement of the right hand.
   Normal response
   (a) Flexion of elbow
   (b) Visible contraction of biceps (Fig. 7.8)
   Abnormal
   (a) Absent—LMN lesion of C5
   (b) Brisk—UMN lesion above C5
   (c) Inverted—Cord lesion C5
2. *Supinator reflex* (*C6*, C5, through radial N)
   (a) Place the arm flexed on the abdomen.
   Place the examiner's index finger 5 cm proximal to the wrist and gently hit the examiner's finger with the percussion hammer.
   Normal response
   (a) Flexion of the elbow visible and contraction of the brachioradialis muscle.
   Abnormal

(a) Absent—LMN lesion of C6
(b) Brisk—UMN lesion above C6
(c) Inverted—cord lesion C6 (Fig. 7.9)

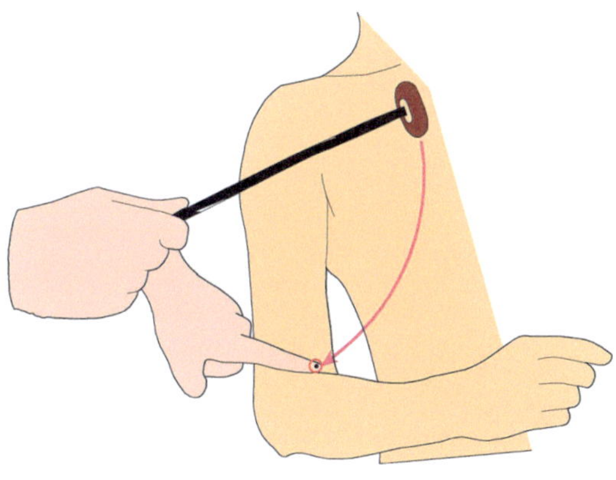

Fig. 7.8 Biceps reflex (C5)

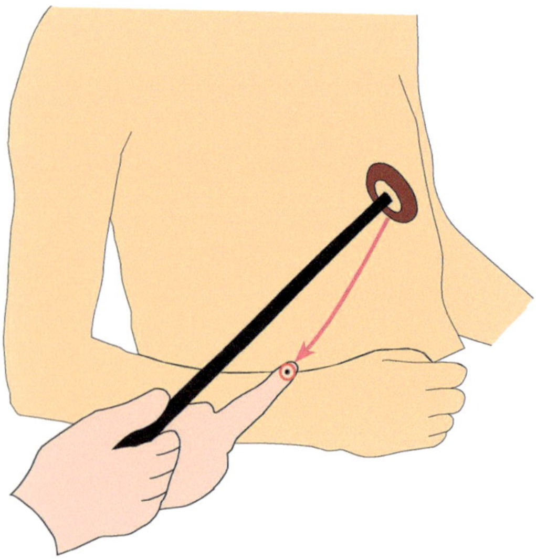

Fig. 7.9 Supinator reflex (C6)

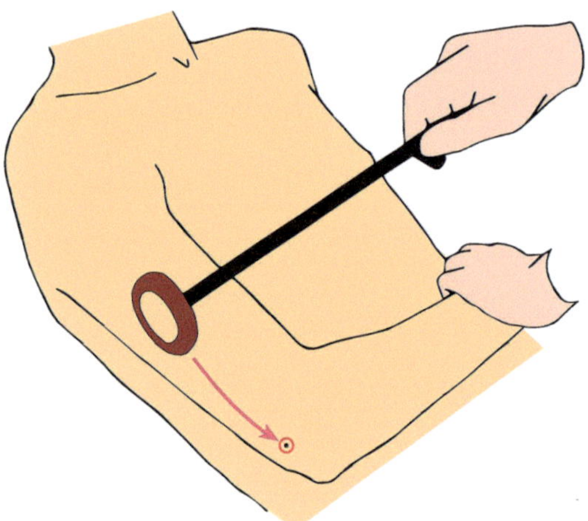

Fig. 7.10 Triceps reflex (C7) (L3)

3. Triceps reflex (C7, though radial N)
   (a) Draw the arm further across the abdomen, holding the wrist with the elbow of the patient at 90° and strike directly the triceps tendon with the hammer.
   Normal response
   (a) Extension of elbow
   (b) Visible contraction of triceps
   Abnormal response
   (c) Absent—LMN C7
   (d) Brisk—UMN lesion above C7 (Fig. 7.10)
4. *Finger flexion* (C8 through ulnar and median nerve)
   (a) Hold the patient's hand in a neutral position with gentle flexion of interphalangeal joint.
   (b) Strike the ball of the examiner's finger.
   Normal response—flexion of fingers
   Abnormal response
   (a) Absent: C8 LMN lesion
   (b) Brisk: UMN lesion above C8
5. *Knee reflex* (*L3* (L4) through femoral N)
   (a) Place the examiner's left arm below both knees of the patient with gentle flexion of both knees to 90°.
   (b) Strike with percussion hammer below the patella.
   Normal response
   (a) Knee extension
   (b) Visible contraction of quadriceps
   Abnormal—absent—L3 LMN lesion
   Brisk—UMN—UMN above L3
   Clonus
   To elicit clonus—hold the patella and pull it downward. Clonus will result in repetitive contractions and up and down movement of the patella (>3 movements) and is indicative of a brisk reflex (Figs. 7.11 and 7.12).
6. *Ankle reflex* (*S1*, (S2), through posterior tibial N)
   (a) Patient's leg is externally rotated with slight flexion at knee.
   (b) Foot is slightly dorsiflexed and the Achilles tendon is hit with the percussion hemmer.
   Normal response
   (a) Plantar flexion of foot.
   (b) Visible contraction of calf muscles.
   Abnormal response
   (a) Absent—LMN lesion S1
   (b) Brisk—UMN lesion above S1 (Fig. 7.13)
   (c) Clonus—To elicit ankle clonus the foot is forcefully dorsiflexed and held in that position. >3 or more contractions resulting in plantar flexion and contraction of the calf muscles is defined as clonus and is indicative of a brisk reflex (Fig. 7.14).

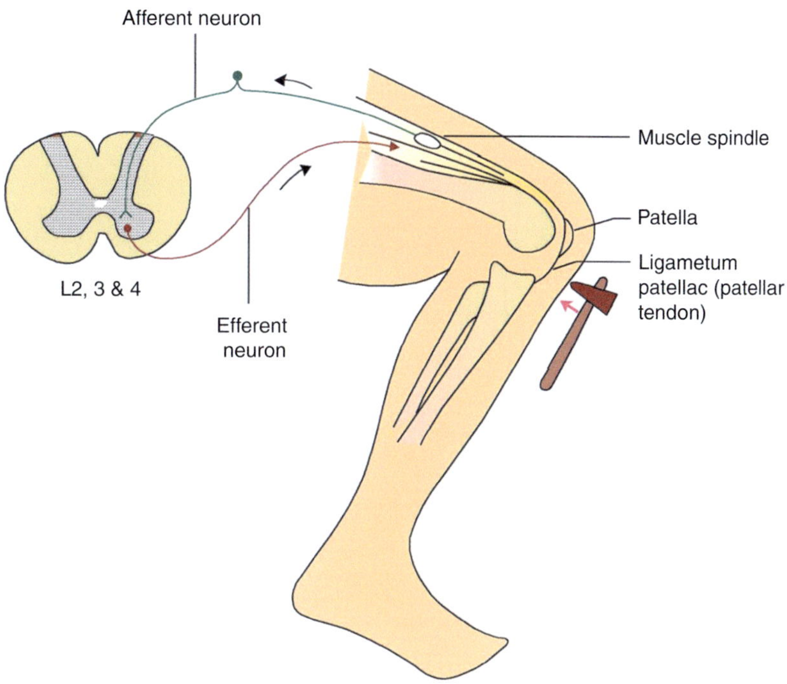

Fig. 7.11 Knee jerk (L3)

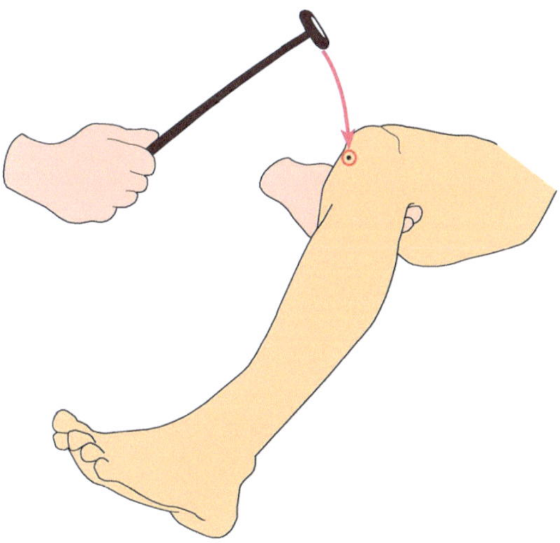

Fig. 7.12 Knee jerk (L3)

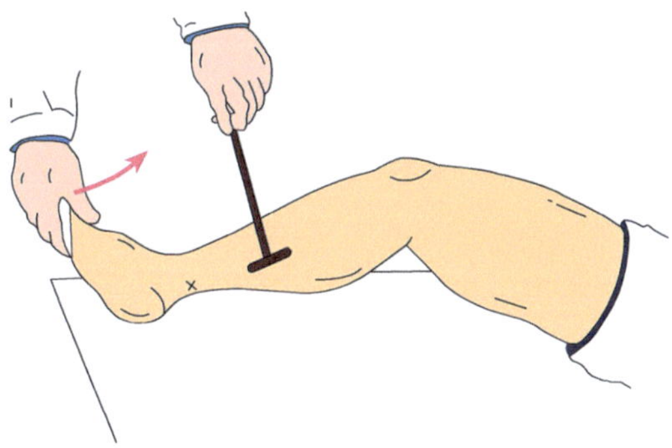

Fig. 7.13 Ankle jerk (S1)

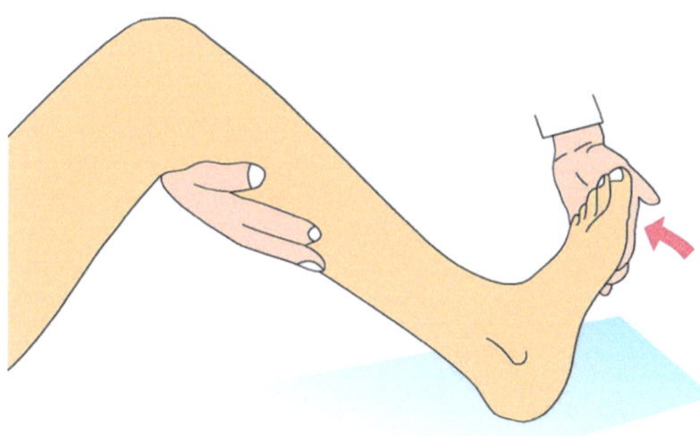

Fig. 7.14 Eliciting ankle clonus

8 Sensory System Examination

The major categories of sensory modalities to be evaluated include:

1. Exteroceptive sensations
2. Proprioceptive sensations
3. Cortical sensations

	Fiber	Tract
(a) Exteroceptive sensations • Pain • Temperature	Small fibers—myelinated and unmyelinated	Spinothalamic tract
(b) Proprioceptive sensations • Vibration • Light touch • Joint position	Large fibers (myelinated)	Posterior column
(c) Cortical sensations • Stereognosis • Two point discrimination • Sensory inattention • Localization of touch • Graphesthesia		Appreciated in thalamus and post-central gyrus

8.1 Exteroceptive Sensations

First-order neurons (small fibers both myelinated and unmyelinated) carry the sensation of pain and temperature from the appropriate receptors and synapse in the dorsal root ganglion. The axons of the second-order neurons cross over to the contralateral side at the same spinal cord level or 1–2 segments above and travel in the lateral and anterior spinothalamic tracts to the ventrolateral nucleus of the thalamus and then project to the post-central gyrus parietal area 3, 1, 2. In the lateral spinothalamic tract the lower part of the body is represented laterally (Fig. 8.1).

8.2 Proprioceptive Sensations

Peripheral axons carry proprioceptive impulses from the skin, spindles, and tendons and these large myelinated fibers continue in the spinal cord and run immediately ipsilaterally in the posterior column to synapse in the Nucleus Gracilis (medial) and Nucleus Cuneatus (lateral) situated at the cervico-medullary junction. Second-order axons from here cross to the contralateral side into the medial laminiscus. And travel in the brainstem till the thalamus. Third-order neurons travel from the thalamus through the posterior limb of internal capsule to reach the post-central gyrus (area 3, 1, 2,). In the posterior column lower part of the body is represented mesialy (Fig. 8.2).

V. Suri, *Clinical Neurological Examination and Localization*,
https://doi.org/10.1007/978-981-16-1228-2_8

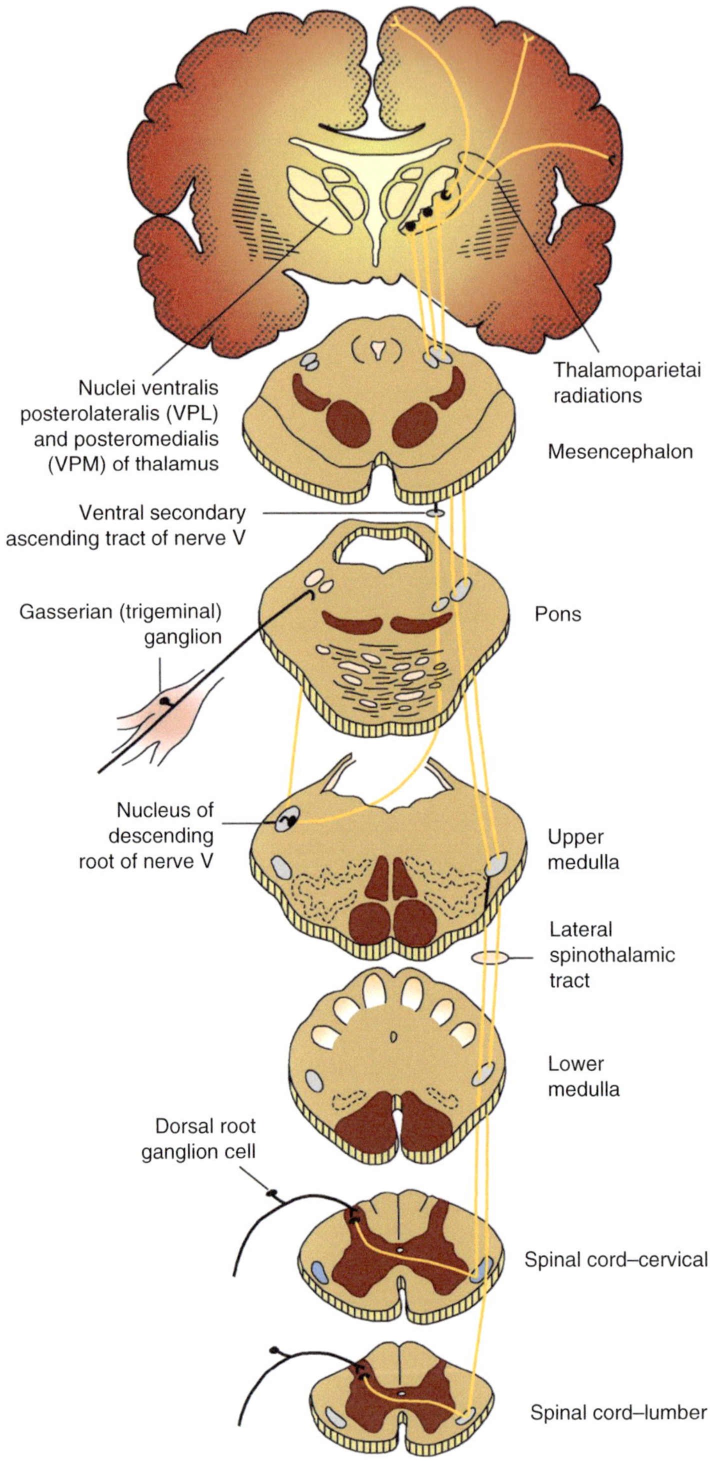

Fig 8.1. The lateral spinothalamic tract

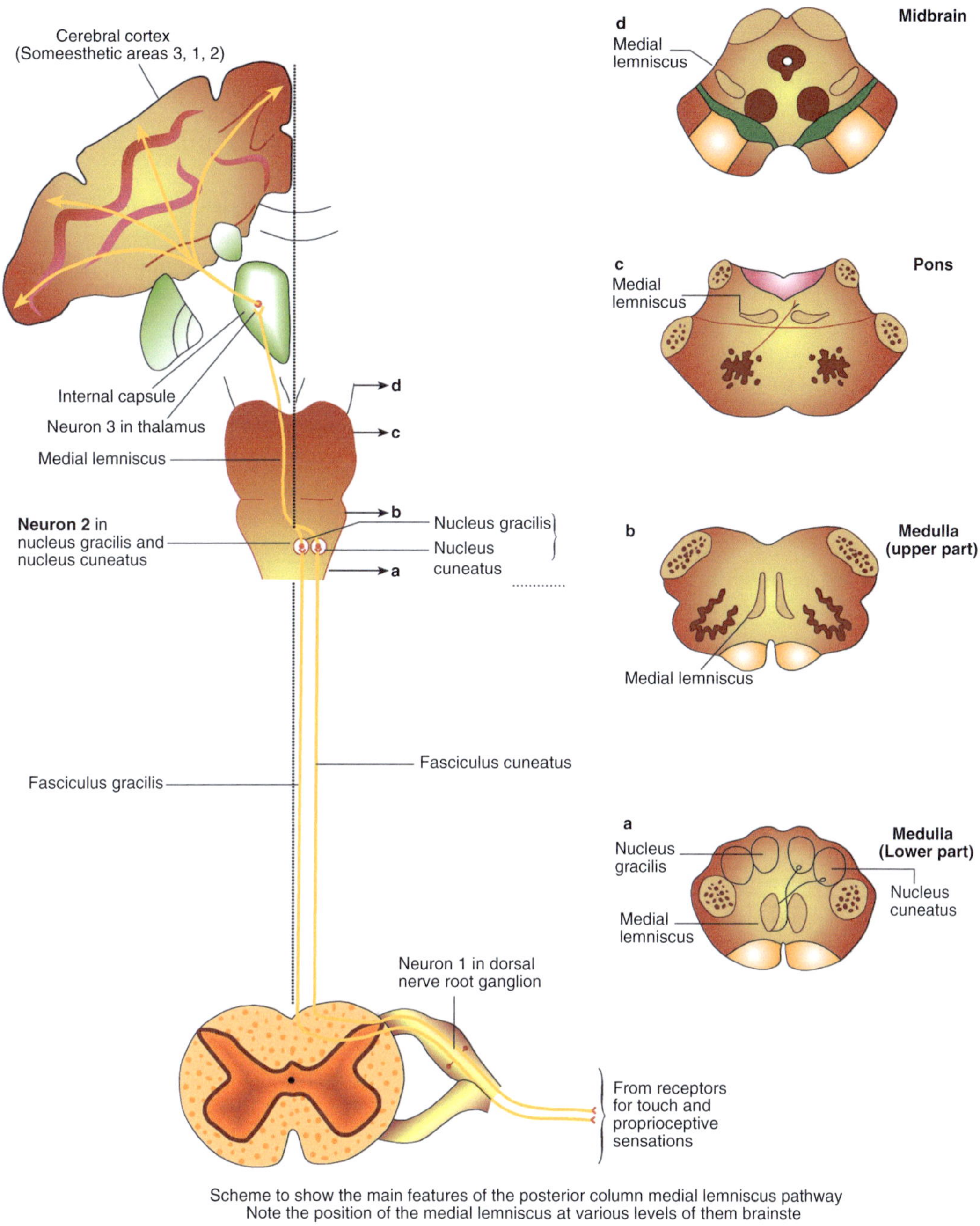

Fig 8.2 Posterior Column pathway

The sensory abnormalities identified should be patterned into various subtypes based on the *distribution of the sensory loss*:

1. Central patterns
   (a) Hemisensory sensory loss (face, trunk, and limbs on one side of the body) (Seen in lesions of post-central gyrus, internal capsule, thalamus).
   (b) Ipsilateral face and contralateral hemisensory loss (Seen in lesion of lateral medulla).
2. Cord
   (a) Sensory levels of exteroceptive loss and proprioceptive loss are identified.
   (b) Dissociate anesthesia: Loss of function of the centrally crossing pain and temperature fibers with intact light touch from posterior column is characteristic of a intramedullary cord lesion, e.g., tumor, syrinx, and trauma.
   (c) Suspended anesthesia: (e.g., hemicape distribution) with normal sensations below and superior to the involved segments. It indicates an intramedullary lesion, e.g., tumor, syrinx, and trauma.
   (d) Sensory loss from the spinal cord segments does not correspond to the same number of vertebrae.

      Upper cervical cord—correspond to the same vertebra.

      Lower cervical cord—subtract 1 for vertebra, e.g., C7 segmental sensory loss will correspond to C6 vertebra

      Upper dorsal cord D1–D6—subtract 2 for vertebral level

      Lower dorsal cord D7–D12—subtract 3 for vertebral level, e.g., D10 sensory loss will correspond to D7 vertebral level.
3. Root or segmental loss:

   The sensory loss is in dermatomal distribution and is usually accompanied by neurogenic pain in the distribution of the radicle.
4. Nerve distribution
   (a) Single nerve—deficit fits into the distribution of a single nerve.
   (b) Mononeuritis multiplex—deficit indicates the involvement of multiple noncontiguous nerves.
   (c) Polyneuropathy—length-dependent distribution of the deficit with maximal deficit occurring distally with gradual spread to proximal regions, i.e., glove and stocking distribution.
   (d) Some important distributions of peripheral nerve supply to memorize:
      - Lateral $3^{1/2}$ palm—median nerve
      - Mesial $1^{1/2}$ palm—ulnar nerve
      - Anatomic snuff box—radial nerve
      - Dorsum of fingers—radial nerve
      - Lateral aspect arm over deltoid—axillary nerve
      - Anterolateral thigh (pocket area)—lateral cutaneous nerve of thigh
      - Anterio-mesial thigh and leg—femoral nerve
      - Posterior thigh, posterior leg, and plantar aspect of sole—sciatic nerve
      - Anterolateral leg and dorsum of foot sparing lateral 2 toes—common peroneal
      - Posterior aspect of leg and sole—posterior tibial nerve

8.2.1 Pain and Temperature Pathway

8.2.1.1 Segmental Sensory Dermatomes

- *C1* no sensory supply on skin
- C2 anterior part of forehead and vertex is supplied by Trigeminal nerve up to the intermeatal line on the vertex and posterior part behind the intermeatal line is supplied by C2
- C4 collar area

- C5 shoulder area
- C6 lateral arm and forearm and lateral fingers and thumb
- C7 posterior arm and forearm running into the middle finger
- C8 T1 mesial forearm and arm and hand
- T4 nipple level
- T6 costal margin
- T10 umblicus
- T12 inguinal ligament region
- L1, L2 L3 anterior thigh
- L4 anterior and mesial leg
- L5 anterior and lateral leg, Great toe
- S1 Little toe and posterior aspect of leg and thigh and heel
- S3–5 Perianal region (Figs. 8.3, 8.4, 8.5, 8.6)

8.2.2 Sensory Areas According to Peripheral Nerves

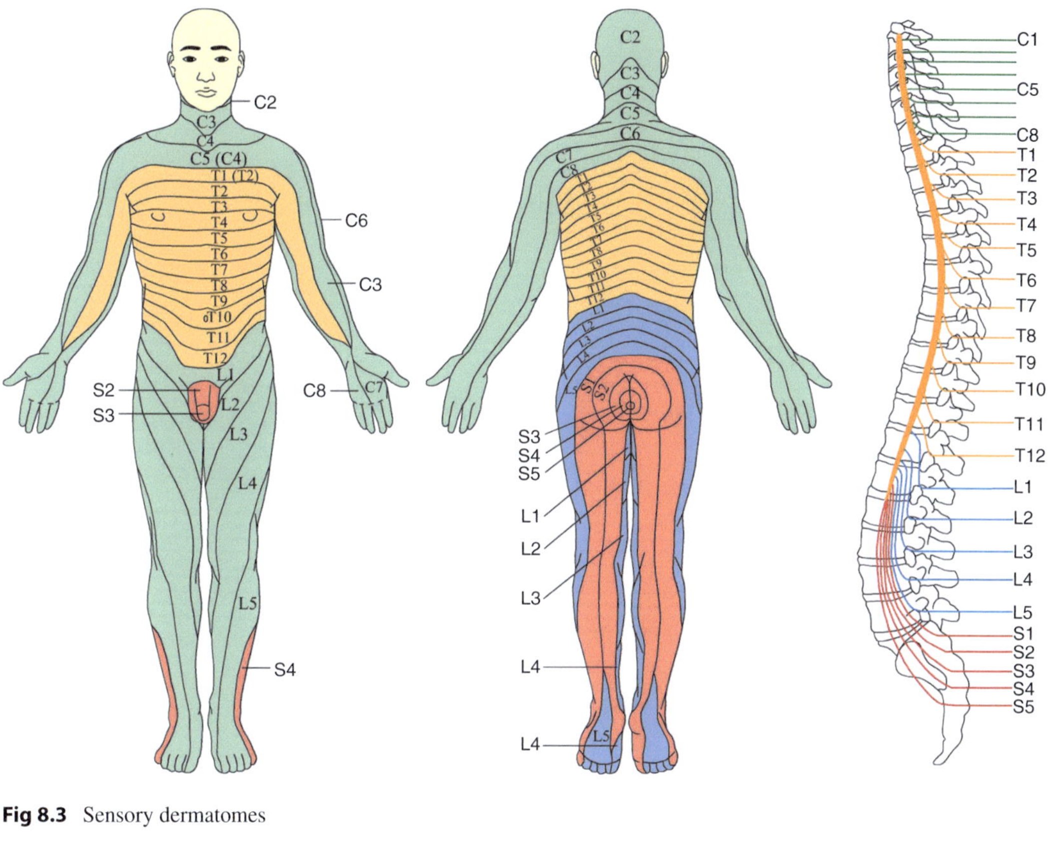

Fig 8.3 Sensory dermatomes

8.2.3 Sensory Loss Patterns

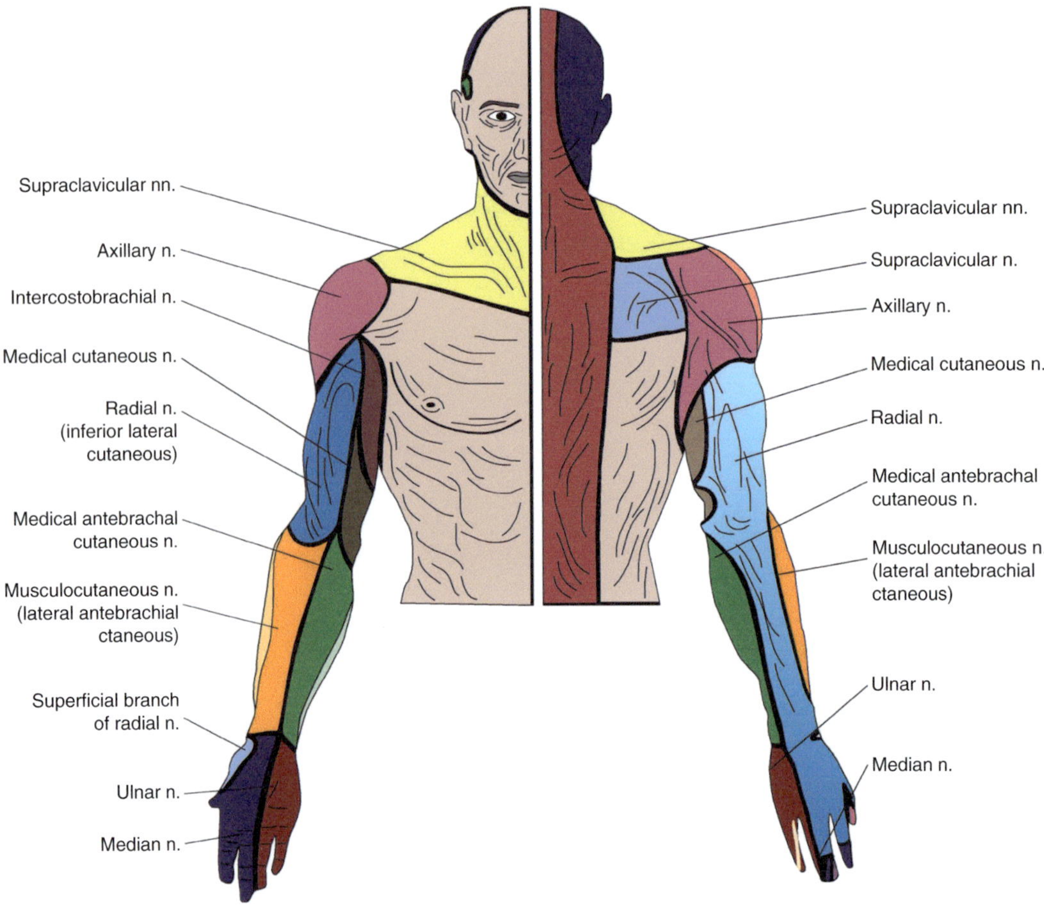

Fig. 8.4 Neural sensory supply of upper limbs

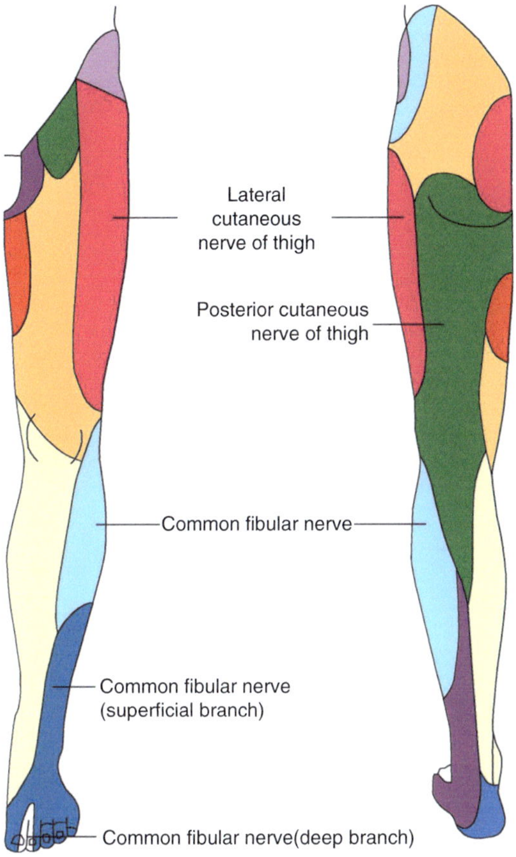

Fig. 8.5 Neural sensory supply of lower limbs

8.3 Clinical Testing

Note: Always test sensations from abnormal zone to normal zone.

1. Light touch
   (a) Dab the patient's skin with a cotton wool wisp or by the examiner's finger. Do not drag the stimulus, e.g., the cotton wisp since that can induce another type of stimulus, i.e., tickling.
   (b) Assess whether the touch is appreciated and whether it is similar in intensity to corresponding areas on the other half of the body and from other body parts.
   (c) Ask the patient with closed eyes to count further every time the patient appreciates a touch and randomly touch at various body parts.
2. Vibration
   (a) Use a *128-Hz* tuning fork. Demonstrate the feel of the vibrating and nonvibrating fork to the patient and ensure that the patient can differentiate between the vibrating and the non-vibrating tuning fork.
   (b) Ask the patient to close eyes and stimulate using a noiselessly vibrating tuning fork starting distally from toes and then moving proximally by stimulating on bony prominences—medial malleolus, tibial tuberosity, anterior iliac spine in lower limb and finger tips, interphalangeal joint, metacarpo-phalangeal joint, wrist, elbow, and shoulder in upper limbs and spinous processes on the spine.
   (c) Patient has to tell whether he/she can feel the vibration and should be able to correctly identify immediately as the vibration ceases. Should assess whether the cessation of the vibration is appropriately felt by evaluating the vibration fork on the examiner's bony prominence after the patient informs cessation of sensation of the vibration.
3. Joint position sense:
   (a) Inform the patient about the test and then ask the patient to close their eyes.
   (b) The distal phalanx of the big toe or other foot toes or thumb and individual fingers in the upper limb are held between the examiner's thumb and index finger at 90° to the intended movement. Ask the patient to inform as soon as the movement is appreciated and whether it is an upward or downward movement.
   (c) Testing is proceeded in a distal to proximal fashion. Upper limbs—interphalangeal joint, metacarpo-phalangeal joint,

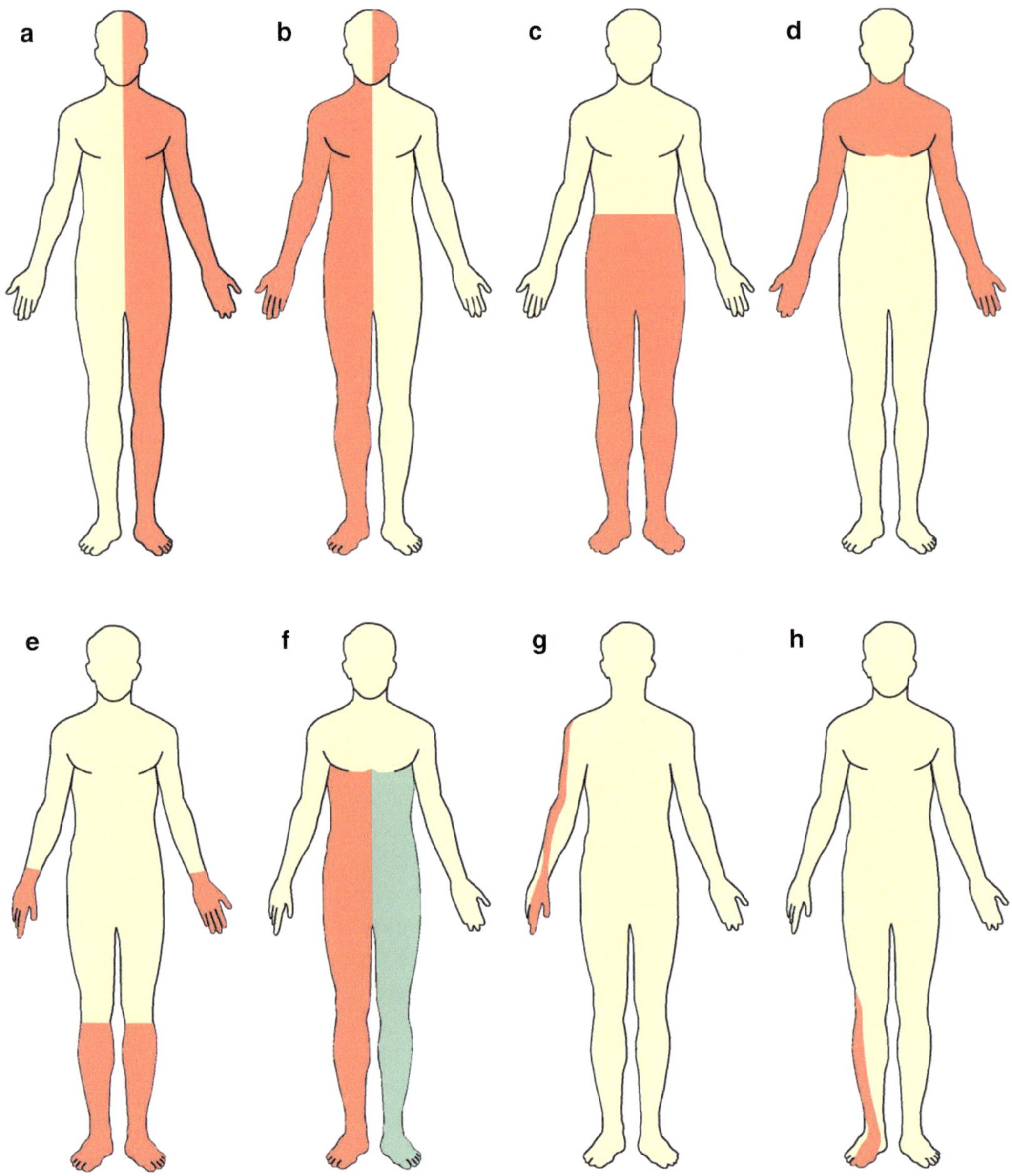

A. Hemisensory loss due to a hemispheric lesion.
B. Crossed sensory loss of pain and temperature due to a lateral medullary lesion.
C. Middorsal spinal cord lesion.
D. Suspended, dissociated sensory loss of pain and temperature due to intramedullary lesion.
E. Distal, symmetric snsory loss due to peripheral neuropathy.
F. Crossed spinothalamic loss on one side with posterior column loss on the opposite side due to hemicord lesion - Brown-Sequard syndrome.
G. Dermatomal sensory loss due to cervical radiculopathy.
H. Dermatomal sensory loss due to lumbosacral radiculopathy.

Fig 8.6 Some common patterns of sensory loss

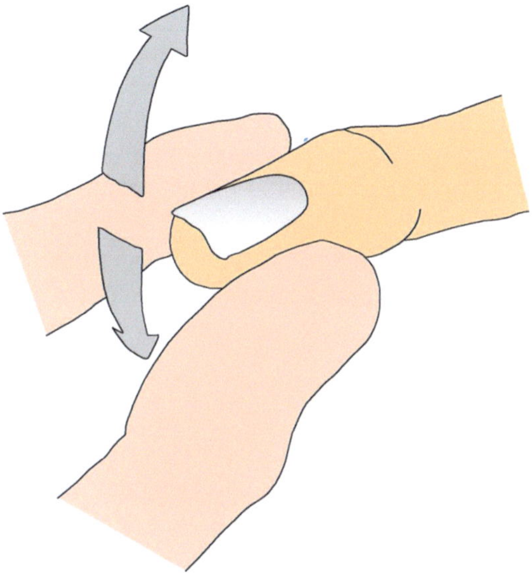

Fig 8.7 Evaluating joint position sense

wrist, elbow, shoulder. Lower limbs—inter phalangeal joint, metatarso-phalangeal joint, ankle, knees, and hip.

(d) A normal response is when a movement of 15°–20° is appreciated at the big toe or thumb (Fig. 8.7).

4. Pain (pin prick) sensation:
   (a) With eyes closed patient is stimulated with a sharp (sharp end of pin, rolling pin) or a blunt object (blunt end of pin) and the patient has to inform the type of sensation felt (sharp or blunt).

   Alternatively a rolling pin-wheel may also be utilized for testing for pain sensation.

   (b) Usually performed from distal to proximal and evaluate for any sharp sensory levels of deficit (and especially for any hyperesthetic band at the level of the sensory loss, which corresponds to the level of the spinal cord lesion).
5. Temperature:
   (a) Two test tubes with cold water (30 °c) and warm water (44 °c) (7 °c below and above 37 °c) are used. Patient is made to appreciate the difference in the temperature by touching on normal skin. Patient then closes his/her eyes and identifies whether the sensation felt is cold or warm.
   (b) Distal to proximal path is followed for testing (alternately abnormal to normal pathway is followed).
6. Cortical sensations:

   Ensure normal light touch before proceeding for cortical sensation evaluation.

   Abnormal cortical sensations indicate parietal lobe (area 3, 1, 2) dysfunction or involvement of parieto-thalamic sensory fibers.

   (a) Stereognosis

   Patients should be able to visually identify the objects. Patient then closes eyes and one object is placed in the hand which the patient has to feel and identify by feeling its texture, shape, and weight.

   (b) Graphesthesia
      I. Numbers are written on the patient's skin using a blunt object. Simple numbers, e.g., 1, 3, 0 that do not involve raising the stimulating stimulus are used. Ensure normal light touch prior to testing. Smaller size letters can be identified on distal sensitive areas, e.g., palm than on lesser sensitive proximal areas, e.g., arm or back.
      II. Size of the letter identified varies from more sensitive to lesser sensitive skin areas. For example, letters of 1–2 mm are identified on the fingertips and 4–6 mm letters are identified over the arm and legs.

   (c) Tactile localization:

   Patient is touched at any body part (with closed eyes) and the patient has to indicate which body part has been touched with exact localization.

   (d) Two point discrimination:
      I. With eyes closed patient is randomly touched with one stimulus or simultaneously two stimuli with the open two point discriminator. Should start the test with two point discriminator wide apart and then gradually reducing the distance between the two points with an aim to identify the

threshold at which the patient cannot differentiate between a single or two point stimulus.

II. Normal two point discrimination varies at different parts with certain sensitive areas allowing discrimination at much smaller distances. Two point discrimination occurs at 2–4 mm at fingertip, 4–6 mm at dorsum and palmar aspect of proximal finger, 8–10 mm on palm, and 2–3 cm on dorsum of the hand.

(e) Sensory inattention

Patient keeps eyes closed, and is stimulated after explanation about the test. Patient is stimulated with light touch stimulation either on one limb or simultaneously on similar points on both limbs. Ability to identify individual touch stimulation but the inability to indicate bilateral simultaneous stimulation is suggestive of the presence of sensory inattention.

9 Cerebellar Examination and Examination of Posture, Stance, and Gait

Coordination is under dominant cerebellar control with some influence from the extrapyramidal system, motor, and sensory systems (especially proprioception).

The cerebellum is divided into certain functional parts with specific nuclei, connections, and function.

Functional classification	Anatomical areas	Nucleus	Major connections	Function
Vestibulocerebellum (archicerebellum)	Floculo-nodular lobe and lingula	Nucleus Fastigius	Vestibular nucleus	Maintains equilibrium in response to labyrinthine stimuli
Paleocerebellum	Whole of anterior lobe (except lingula, uvula, and pyramid)	Nucleus emboliform and nucleus globose	Spinal cord	Maintaining tone and crude control of movement
Neocerebellum	Whole of posterior lobe (except pyramid and uvula)	Nucleus dentate	Pons	Coordination of skilled voluntary movement

9.1 Cerebellar Signs

9.1.1 Vermian

- Truncal ataxia with tendency to fall backward or forward.
- Titubition
- Ataxia dysarthria

9.1.2 Hemispherical cerebellar signs

- Nystagmus
- Dysmetria (finger-nose, knee-skin-heel)
- Hypotonia
- Intention tremor
- Ataxia with tendency to reel toward the ipsilateral side

9.2 Clinical Tests

9.2.1 Dysmetria

Impaired limb coordination manifesting as under-shooting or over-shooting the target.

V. Suri, *Clinical Neurological Examination and Localization*,
https://doi.org/10.1007/978-981-16-1228-2_9

9.2.1.1 Finger–Nose Test

Patient is asked to touch the tip of the examiner's index finger (kept at a distance so that patient's arm is fully extended to reach it) and smoothly take it back and forth between the tip of his/her nose and the examiner's index finger. The test is then repeated with eyes closed (marked worsening will indicate proprioception loss).

The test is then repeated on the opposite upper limb.

Observe for under or overshooting and crudeness of movement. It indicates Dysmetria in the upper limb and results from ipsilateral cerebellar hemispherical lesions (Fig. 9.1).

9.2.1.2 Knee-Skin-Heel Test

- In lying down position, patient runs his/her heel of one leg on the opposite side shin from knee downward to the anterior foot followed by raising the heel and repeating the test from knee downward. It is then repeated with the other leg. Observe for side to side veering of the heel away from the shin which indicates dysmetria and it indicates a lesion of the ipsilateral cerebellum.
- The test is repeated with eyes closed (for proprioception loss) (Fig. 9.2).

9.2.2 Dysdiadokokinesia

- Patient sits with arms flexed at elbow and holding the forearms forward, parallel to the floor. Patient then rotates both hands at the wrist as if "screwing or unscrewing a nut." Observe for crudeness and slow and irregular movement on any one or both sides.
- Can evaluate also by rapidly and alternatingly placing the palm followed by the dorsum of one hand on the palm of the other hand and observe for errors and slowing and clumsiness of the movement.
- Abnormal in lesions of ipsilateral cerebellum.

9.2.3 Titubation

Titubation is a slow (3–4 Hz) usually anterior to posterior ("yes–yes") oscillatory movement of the head. Occasionally, the head movement is side to side ("No–No"). This is seen in lesions of the cerebellar vermis.

9.2.4 Intention tremor

Slow, action tremor usually precipitated and aggravated by performing the finger–nose test

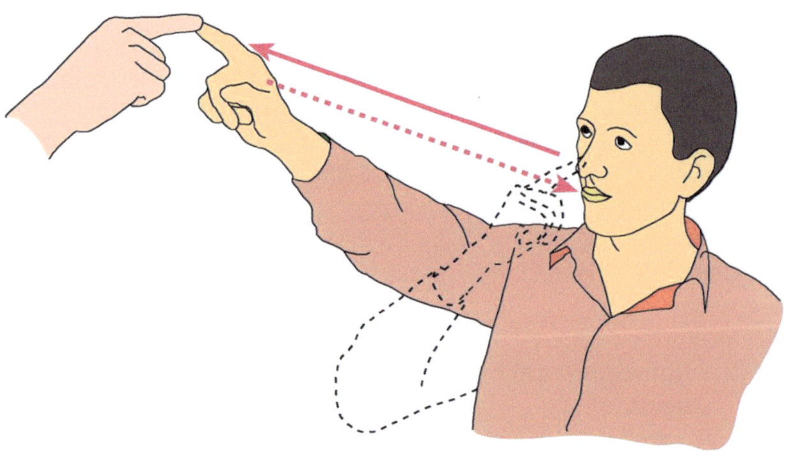

Fig. 9.1 Finger nose test—dysmetria in upper limbs

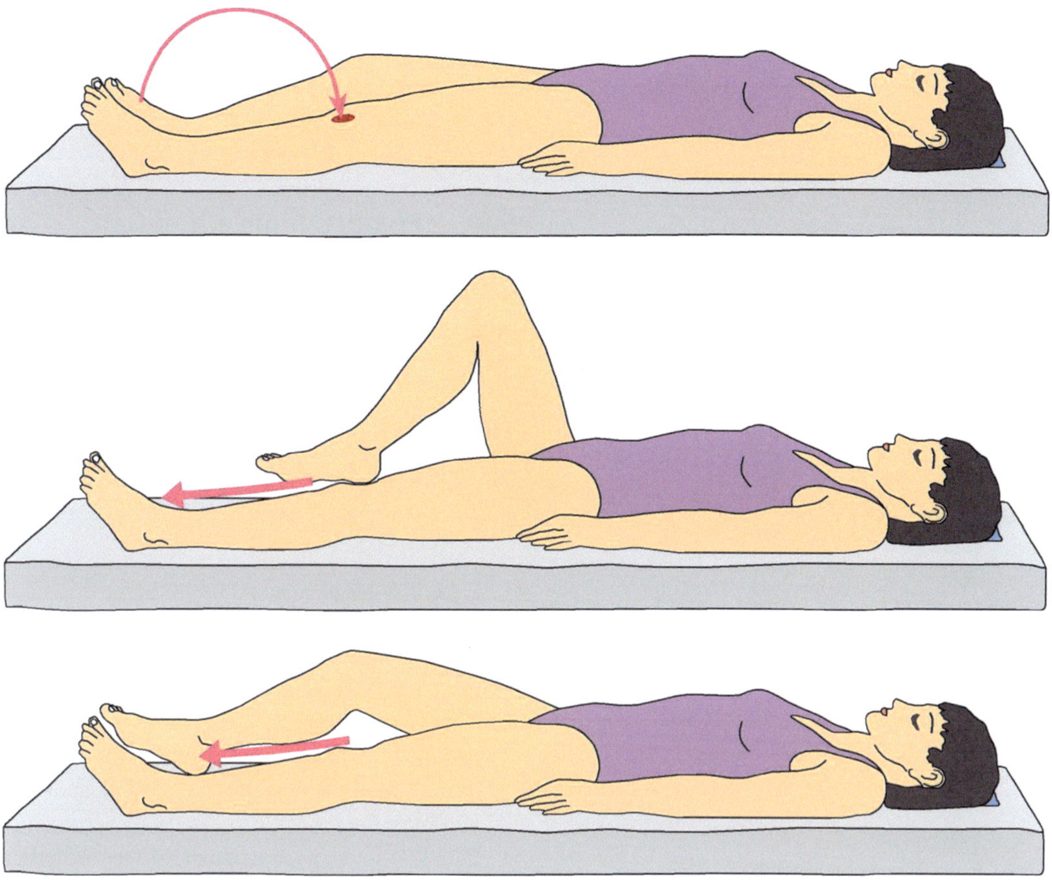

Fig. 9.2 Heel knee shin test—dysmetria in lower limbs

with tremor showing marked worsening on approaching close to the target. It is seen in ipsilateral limbs in cerebellar hemispherical lesions.

9.2.5 Truncal Ataxia

Patients with hemispherical cerebellar dysfunction have unsteadiness and walk on a broad base with tendency to veer to the side of the cerebellar lesion. Subtle abnormalities can be assessed by asking the patient to walk in Tandem, i.e., walk in a straight line while touching the toes of one foot with the heel of the front foot (Fig. 9.3).

9.2.6 Pendular Knee Jerk

Patient is made to sit on a chair with the legs dangling and few inches above the ground and the patella is struck with the percussion hammer to elicit the knee jerk. oscillations more than two and a half indicate a pendular knee jerk and indicate ipsilateral cerebellar dysfunction.

9.2.7 Holmes Rebound phenomenon

Patient stands and keeps both the arms flexed at the elbow. Examiner applies force to extend the arms and informs the patient that he/she will sud-

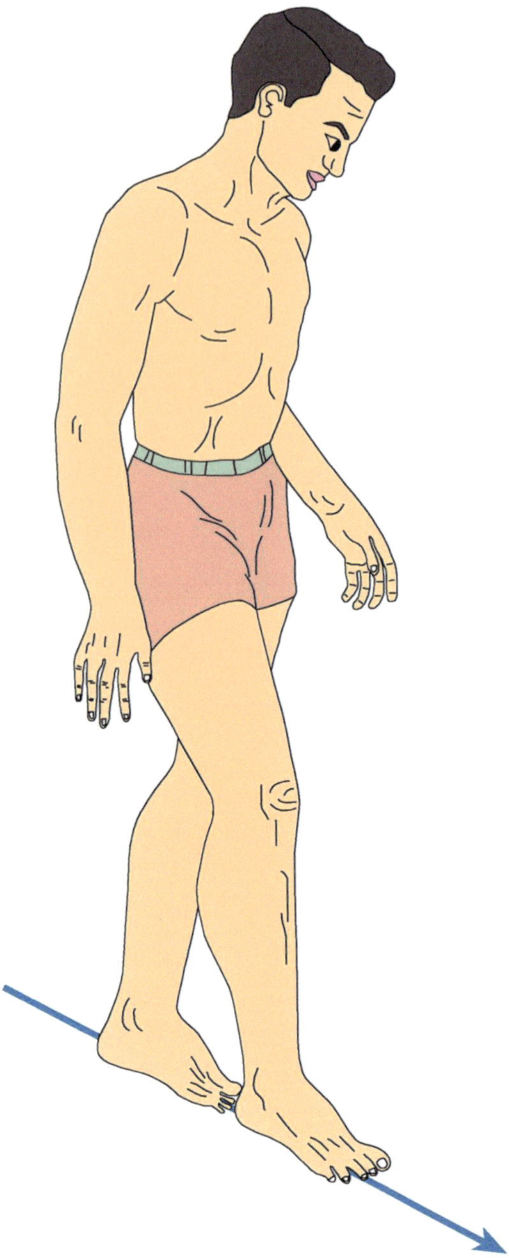

Fig. 9.3 Tandem walk for truncal ataxia

denly stop applying force on the patient's arm. The patient's arm on the abnormal side cannot be controlled and will flex back in a uncontrollable manner (Fig. 9.4).

9.2.8 Hypotonia

Loss of tone maybe elicited ipsilateral to the cerebellar lesion.

9.3 Posture, Stance, and Gait

Posture of the patient while standing and the gait while walking is an important and essential evaluation, which is frequently conducted in outpatients but erroneously missed in admitted patients who are lying in bed.

9.3.1 Posture and Stance

- Patient is asked to stand up in the position he/she normally adopts.
- Next patient is asked to stand with both legs close together (heel and toes touching).
- Next while standing with feet close together patient is asked to close his/her eyes (assure the patient that he/she will not fall and that you have the patient protected).
- Patient is given a gentle push to assess whether the patient is able to maintain posture or has a tendency to fall to either side or backward or forward.

Evaluate for:

1. *Stooped posture*: Seen in Parkinson's disease or old age.
2. *Lordotic posture of trunk*: Seen in trunkal weakness, especially in muscular dystrophies.
3. *Kyphotic or scoliotic deformity of spine*: Seen in neurogenic weakness of trunkal muscles or in skeletal pathology of the spine.
4. *Imbalance on standing*: Patient is unable to stand on a narrow base with feet close together.
   - Cerebellar lesion—Patient cannot stand on a narrow base with tendency to reel toward the side of lesion.

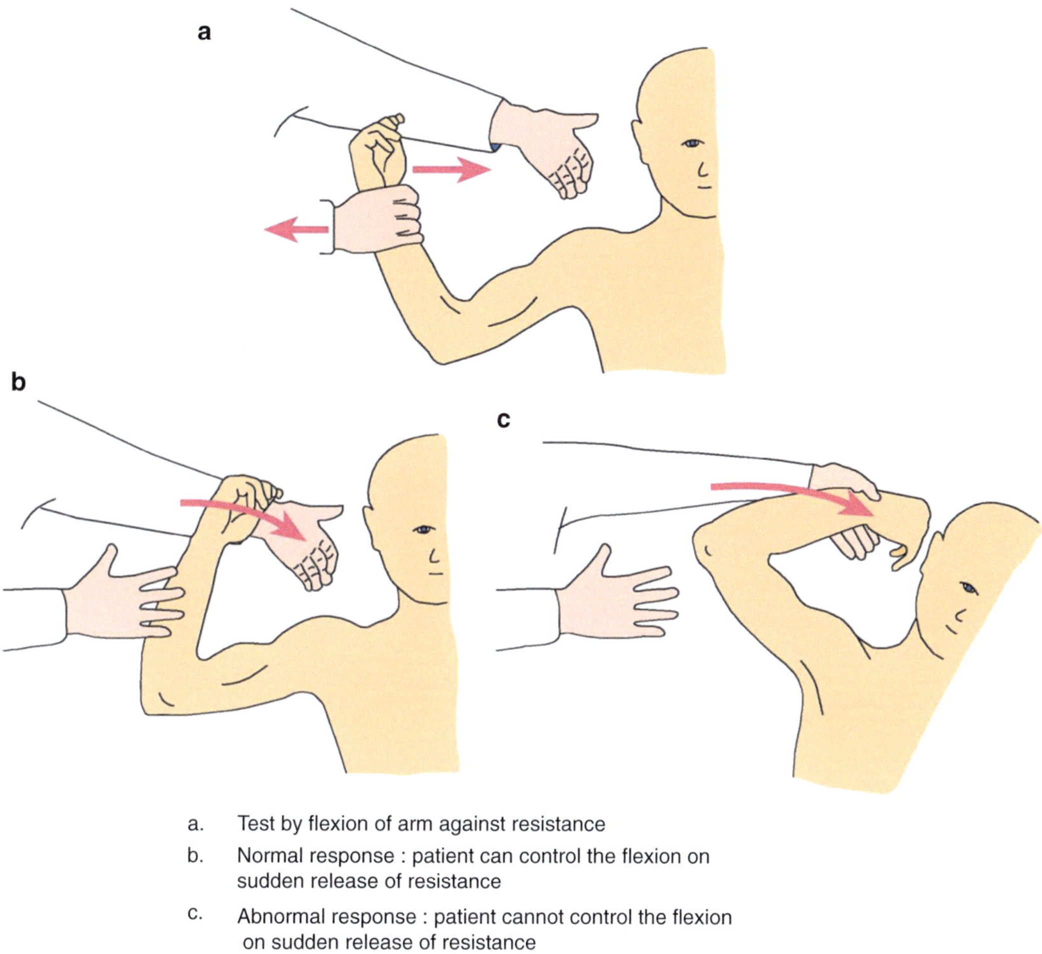

Fig. 9.4 Rebpund phenomenon in cerebellar disease

- Posterior column lesion or sensory ataxia, e.g., subacute combined degeneration of cord, posterior cord lesion, sensory neuropathy. Patient is able to stand with feet close together but has severe veering on immediately closing eyes (Romberg's test positive).

9.3.2 Gait

- Ask the patient to walk normally away from you and then turn and return back.
- Ask the patient next to walk in tandem in a straight line touching the toe of one foot to the heel of the other foot.
- Then check for retropulsion by the *pull back test*. Stand behind the patient after explaining that the patient will be pulled back from his/her shoulder by a gentle push and the patient has to attempt to keep standing and not be pulled or fall backward. Later gradually keep increasing the pull force and the patient has to attempt not to fall backwards and to keep standing firmly.

Normal: patient keeps his/her feet firmly on the floor and adjusts his/her trunk back into place.

Abnormal: patient is pulled backward and takes a few steps backward with tendency to fall backward (retropulsion). Seen in patients with Parkinson's plus syndrome.

Observe the Gait for the following features:

1. Initiation of gait
2. Base—wide or narrow
3. Symmetrical or asymmetrical gait, i.e., involves one side or both sides of the body
4. Stride—small steps or long
5. Turning—any freezing or imbalance
6. Speed of movement—slow or fast
7. Associated arm movements
8. Balance—tendency to reel to any particular side or retropulsion (backward)
9. Pull test—check for retropulsion

Evaluate for:

1. *Asymmetrical gait abnormality* involving one leg, e.g., hemiplegia (UMN), or radiculopathy or neuropathy (LMN) vs. symmetrical gait abnormality involving both legs and truncal balance.
2. *Symmetrical gait abnormality* with abnormality of balance of bilateral limbs.
3. Check for *narrow based vs. broad based* gait
   (a) Narrow based—
      (i) Parkinson's
      (ii) Frontal lobe ataxia
      (iii) Normal pressure hydrocephalus
   (b) Broad based
      (i) Cerebellar pathology
      (ii) Sensory ataxia (posterior column lesion, subacute combined degeneration of cord, sensory neuropathy)
      (iii) Mild broad based with prominent waddling (falling of pelvis) in patients with proximal muscle weakness, e.g., in muscular dystrophies.

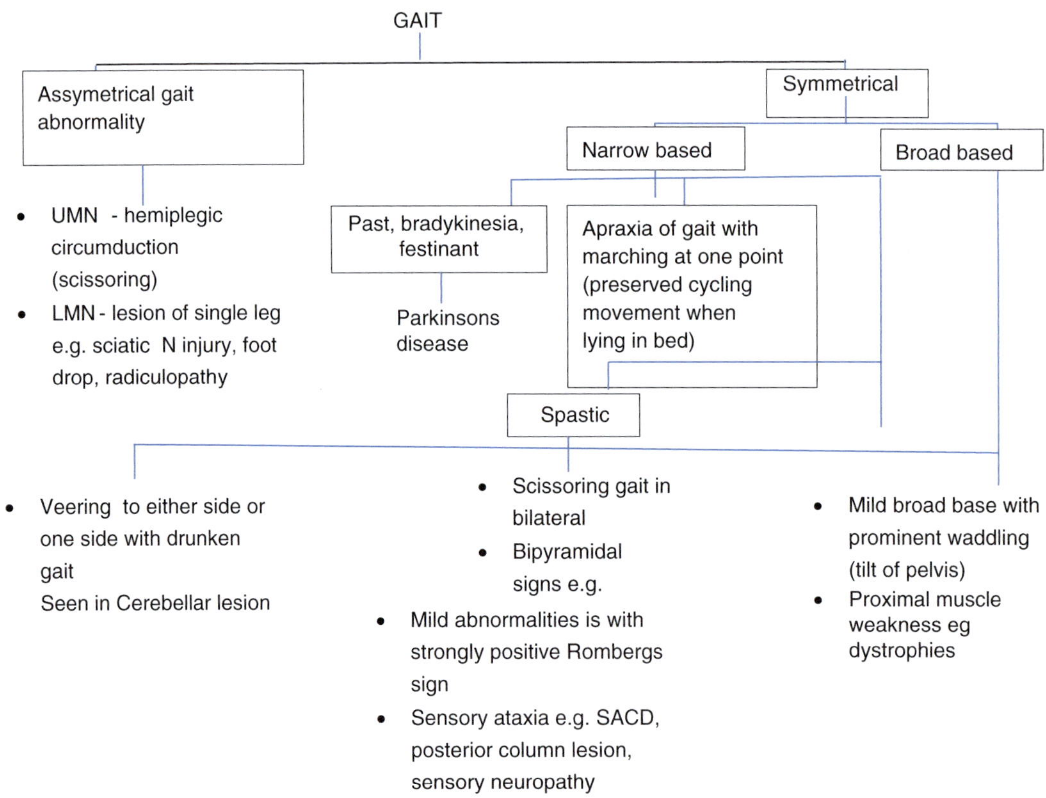

GAIT

9.4 Common Gait Disorders

9.4.1 Asymmetrical Gait

9.4.1.1 Hemiplegic Gait

Circumduction of the paralyzed leg with dragging of the foot. Arm is adducted, flexed at the elbow, and pronated and flexed at the wrist.

9.4.1.2 Foot Drop

Patient takes a high step on the paralyzed leg with a loud slapping audible sound.

9.4.2 Symmetrical Gait

9.4.2.1 Apraxic Gait

Difficulty in the initiation of gait followed by short shuffling and tendency to march at one spot. Base may be wide or narrow. Feet seem to be glued to the floor with tendency to freeze on initiation of movements, while passing through narrow spaces and while turning. Patient maybe able to produce significantly preseved cycling or other leg movements while lying in bed. Seen in patients with NPH, frontal lobe dysfunction, and Parkinson's disease.

9.4.2.2 Sensory Ataxia

There is usually gross ataxia with a wide base and tendency of high steppage gait and patient has a tendency to focus on the floor while walking with tendency to fall on closing eyes. Seen in patients with subacute combined degeneration of cord, sensory neuropathies, and posterior cord lesions.

9.4.2.3 Cerebellar Gait

Patient walks on a wide base with irregular foot placement and possibly with titubation and rhythmic truncal and head tremor in patients with pancerebellar syndromes. This simulates a drunken gait. Unilateral cerebellar lesions result in drifting to the side of the lesion.

9.4.2.4 Paraplegic or Quadriplegic Gait

Patient walks slowly with stiff and extended legs and the legs cross each other like a "scissor." Seen in compressive and non-compressive myelopathies, multiple sclerosis, and brainstem lesions.

9.4.2.5 Waddling Gait

Patient walks on a normal or wide base with side to side waddling and tilting of the pelvis. Occurs in patients with proximal muscle weakness.

9.4.2.6 Antalgic Gait

This is a non-neurological gait occurring due to pain in the hip or knee or leg and thigh. Patient avoids weight bearing and may simulate a neurological gait.

10 Involuntary Movements

Movement disorders disrupt motor function, not by weakness but either by reducing the amount of free-flowing movement (labeled as Hypokinetic disorders) or by producing involuntary and undesired movements (labeled as Hyperkinetic disorders). It is important to accurately assess the type of involuntary movement and then assess whether it is an isolated disorder (and ascertain its possible cause) or whether it is part of a neurological syndrome (e.g., rest tremor with other components of Parkinson's disease).

The movement should be identified:

(a) In resting position
(b) While raising both arms in front
(c) In different postures and while initiating movement

It is important to assess:

(a) *Distribution*—Which part is affected?
(b) *Periodicity*—Is the movement paroxysmal or continuous?
(c) *Rhythm*—Is it rhythmic (tremor), arrhythmic (chorea), fast, and slow?
(d) *Relation to postures*—Is the movement present at rest, or in certain postures, e.g., outstretched arms or precipitated by action, e.g., bringing the hand close to the nose. Does it disappear in sleep?
(e) *Speed*—Fast as in myoclonus, intermediate as in tremor or chorea, and slow as in dystonia.
(f) *Relation to sleep*—Is it present during sleep, e.g., myoclonus or palatal tremor. Most movements will disappear during sleep.
(g) *Suppressibility*—Voluntary suppression as in tics, sensory tricks in dystonia, and suppression of rest tremor by activity.
(h) *Relieving factors*—Walking sideways or backward may relieve dystonia and alcohol intake may temporarily relieve action postural tremors.

10.1 Types of Movement Disorders

10.1.1 Hypokinetic Disorders

The prototype of hypokinetic movement disorder is Parkinson's disease with Bradykinesia, rest tremor, cogwheel rigidity, and postural imbalance.

10.1.2 Hyperkinetic Disorders

These include Tremors, Chorea, Athetosis, Tics, Hemiballismus, Dystonia, Tardive Dyskinesias, myoclonus, and Asterixis.

V. Suri, *Clinical Neurological Examination and Localization*,
https://doi.org/10.1007/978-981-16-1228-2_10

10.1.2.1 Tremor

Tremors are rhythmic oscillations of the body part caused by intermittent muscle contractions and are the commonest movement disorder. Tremors are broadly divided into four types:

1. Postural tremor
2. Action tremor
3. Rest tremor
4. Intention tremor

Clinical Testing

- Assess the tremor at rest, with outstretched arms (with a piece of paper placed lightly on the hand), or while doing finger–nose test (postural and intention tremors). One can also assess the tremor by asking the patient to copy the Archimedes spiral, which is extremely important in differentiating action tremor from rest tremor.

Postural Tremor

Evaluated by asking the patient to outstretch both arms and spread the fingers. The tremor can be appreciated better by placing a sheet of paper on the hand and watching its movement.

Action Tremor

Becomes prominent while performing action and hence is the most disabling. The tremor is usually perpendicular to the action and is usually evaluated by asking the patient to perform the finger–nose test.

Action and Postural tremors virtually always coexist although one may be more prominent than the other and hence labeled accordingly. Prototypes of the Action–postural tremor include:

- Physiological tremor—8–12 Hz tremor seen in normal persons with exacerbation by anxiety, anger, certain drugs, and hyperthyroidism.
- Essential tremor—familial action and postural tremor occurring at 8 Hz and especially involving upper limbs and later jaw, head, and speech. It is usually postural tremor and prominent on outstretched arms. It worsens with anxiety and anger and is briefly suppressed with alcohol (Fig. 10.1).

Intention Tremor

Slower, action tremor usually precipitated and aggravated by performing the finger–nose test with tremor worsening on approaching close to the target. Seen in ipsilateral limbs in cerebellar lesions. It affects proximal muscles more than the distal muscles.

Rest Tremor

Rest tremor is a tremor that is most prominent at rest and maybe pill rolling in character and occurs at a slower frequency of 3–7 Hz. It reduces briefly while performing voluntary activity, e.g., raising the arm (will cause transient cessation and will reemerge when the outstretched arm position is maintained). It can be precipitated by asking the

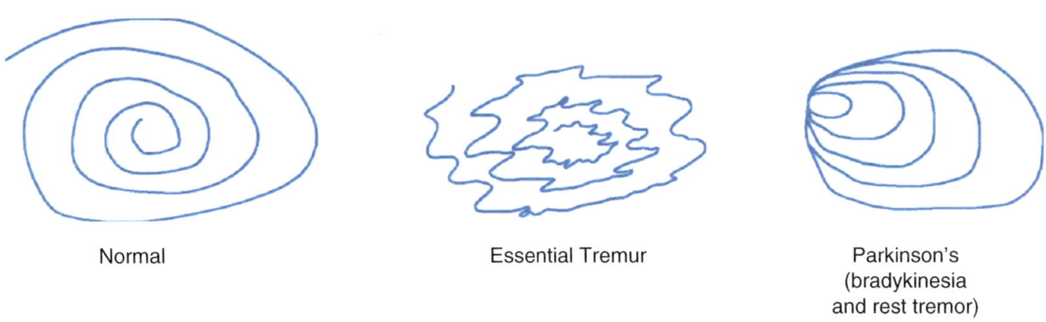

Fig. 10.1 Archimides spiral

patient to keep both hands semi-pronated on the thighs and counting backward from 100.

The Archimedes spiral will usually not reveal the tremor but will reveal evidence of bradykinesia (crowding of lines in one direction).

Certain Other Tremors

- Dystonic tremor—4–8 Hz tremor seen in dystonic muscles on attempting to control the dystonic movement.
- Rubral tremor—seen in patients with lesions of the superior cerebellar peduncle, midbrain tegmentum, or posterior thalamus. This is an irregular, slow 4–5 Hz, large-amplitude tremor occurring at rest with aggravation by sustained posture.
- Primary orthostatic tremor—12–18 Hz tremor involving legs when standing erect. It is considered a type of essential tremor.

10.1.2.2 Chorea

Arrhythmic, nonrepetitive, semi-purposive involuntary and almost continuous, rapid movements involving upper limbs, tongue, or even trunk.

Disorders commonly causing chorea:

1. Huntington chorea (genetic)
2. Sydenham's chorea (streptococcal infections)
3. Neuroacanthocytosis (autosomal recessive with dystonia, tics, and self-mutilation).
4. SLE

10.1.2.3 Athetosis

Slower, arrhythmic, writhing movement of hand, wrist, and arms with dominant involvement of distal muscles.

- Seen in patients with Wilson's disease, cerebral palsy, and kernicterus.

10.1.2.4 Tics

Stereotyped and irresistible, repetitive movements, and occasionally associated with involuntary sound (vocal tics), and are usually preceded by urge to make the movement with brief relief after completion of the movement.

- Usually affects the face (blinking, grimacing, winking, twitching the nose) neck, shoulder (shrugging), and vocal tics involving sounds, e.g., clearing the throat sound.
- Seen in chronic tic disorder or in Gilles de la Tourette syndrome where there is a combination of motor and vocal tics and coprolalia, and other obsessive traits.

10.1.2.5 Hemi-Ballismus

Violent flinging, unilateral large amplitude, flinging movement of the arm.

- Caused by lesions of the subthalamic nucleus.

10.1.2.6 Dystonia

Sustained or repetitive abnormal muscle contraction with co-contraction of agonist and antagonist muscles leading to abnormal posturing with or without tremor or jerks.

- Can be focal, segmental, or generalized.
- Generalized dystonia's may include primary dystonia of childhood, dopa responsive or Segawa disease, or dystonic forms of Parkinson's disease.
- Focal dystonia's include cervical dystonia, oromandibular dystonia, spasmodic dysphonia, Meig's syndrome, and writer's cramp.

10.1.2.7 Asterixis

Seen by asking the patient to outstretch both arms with dorsiflexed wrists. Patient cannot maintain the posture with repeated involuntary jerk like loss of posture of the upper limbs resulting in dropping of the arms. It is also called negative myoclonus

- Seen in encephalopathies, e.g., hepatic, uremic, or hyponatremic

10.1.2.8 Myoclonus

Sudden, shock like, rapid muscular jerks involving limbs, or trunk. These may be focal, unilateral, or generalized.

- Could be epileptic or arise from various cortical, brain stem, or cord lesions.

10.1.2.9 Tardive Dyskinesias

Multiple types of involuntary movements mainly involving the face, lips, jaw, and tongue.

- Occurring as a complication of usage of dopamine antagonists, e.g., neuroleptic medication and in patients with Parkinson's disease, Wilson's disease, and Sydenham chorea.

11 Examination of Skull, Spine, Nerves, and Neurocutaneous Markers

Examination of the skull, spine, thickened nerves, and presence of any neurocutaneous markers is conducted and documented as a routine at the end of the neurological examination, though a variety of these deformities, e.g., Kyphosis, Scoliosis, or skull abnormalities are already obvious during other previous evaluations.

11.1 Skull

Examine the shape, size of the skull, and evaluate for any bony or soft tissue lumps.

Auscultate the skull for any bruits.

- Hydrocephalus—large head
- Microcephaly—small head, may be associated with mental retardation
- Craniosynostosis—abnormal shapes of the skull
- Acromegaly—large head with elongation with large jaw, ears, and nose
- Basilar invagination—short neck with low hairline and restricted neck movements and head placed in mild extension (Figs. 11.1, 11.2 and 11.3)

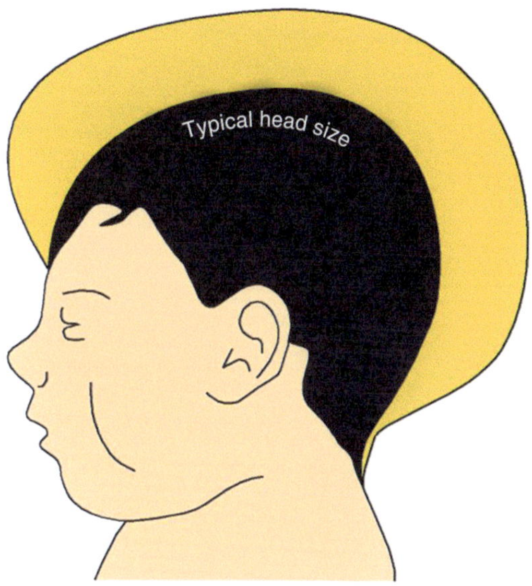

Fig. 11.1 Hydrocephalus

11.2 Spine

Kyphosis—normal convex curvature of the spine occurs in thoracic and sacral regions. A curvature > or = 45° constitutes kyphosis.

Scoliosis—where the spine takes a C or S lateral curve. Any curve >10° is considered abnormal.

- Evaluate for kyphosis or scoliosis and differentiate from neurogenic scoliosis (spine

V. Suri, *Clinical Neurological Examination and Localization*,
https://doi.org/10.1007/978-981-16-1228-2_11

straightens up on forward bending as in touching the feet with both arms) in neurogenic deformity vs. fixed deformity with no straightening in patients with skeletal deformities.

- *Evaluate* for any tuft of hair or dimple at the lower end of the spine which may indicate an occult spinal dysraphism.

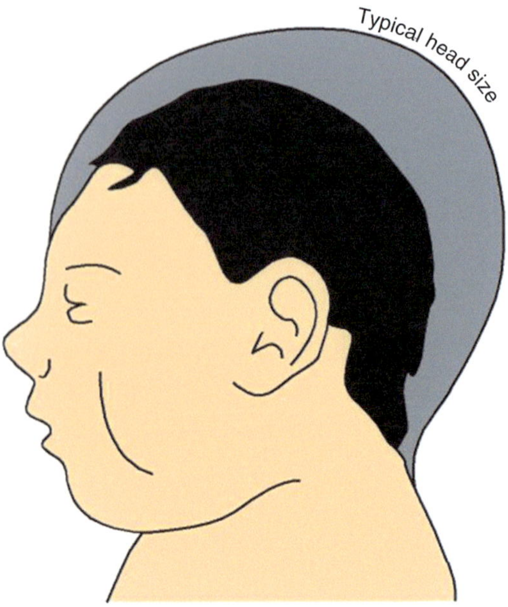

Fig. 11.2 Microcephaly

Short neck is seen in Klippel-feil, Noonan, Turner syndromes, and in patients with cranio-vertebral junction abnormalities.

Neck length is measured by using a Two point discriminator with one point on Inion and the other on the Spinous process of C7 vertebrae.

$$\frac{\text{Body length}}{\text{Inion to C7 length}} = \text{normal} < 13:1$$
$$= \text{abnormal for short neck if ratio is more than } 13:1.$$

Low Hair Line

- Low hair line is labeled when the hair on the neck extends more inferiorly than usual.
- Distance between the hairline (trichion) and the glabella (most prominent part of the frontal bone just above the root of the nose) in the midline is measured and it is abnormal if it is more than 2SD below the mean (Fig. 11.4).

11.3 Thickened Nerves

Inspection and palpation to evaluate for any nerve thickening is conducted. The greater

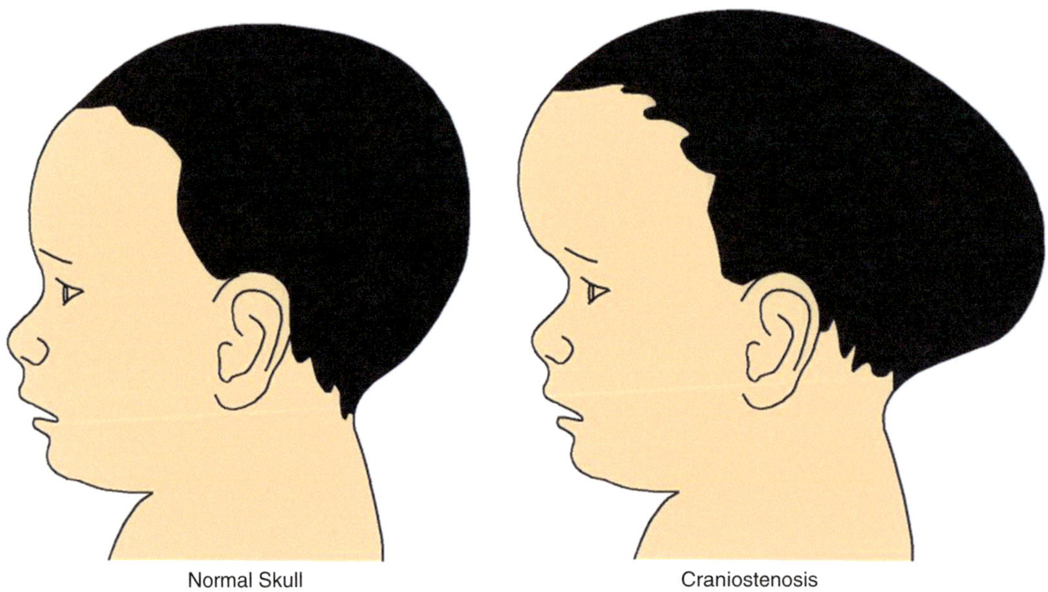

Fig. 11.3 Craniosynostosis

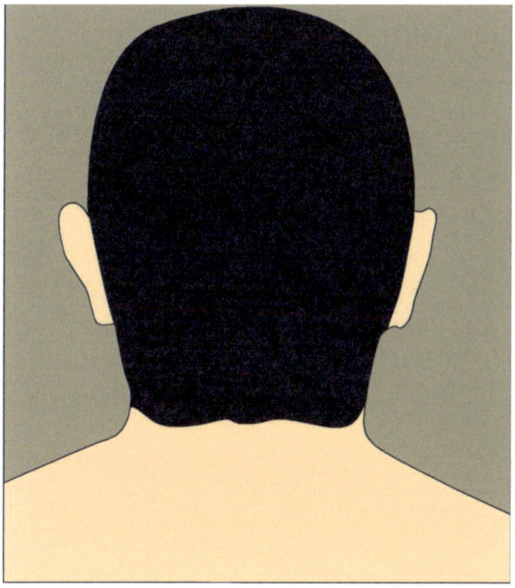

Fig. 11.4 Low hair line

auricular nerve in the neck is commonly thickened in 1 Hansen's disease when it is also associated with thickening of other nerves and dermal patches of hypo-anesthetic lesions with trophic changes.

Other nerves, e.g., median at wrist, radial nerve at wrist, ulnar nerve at elbow, common peroneal nerve at neck of fibula, and sural nerve in posterior leg are palpated for any thickening (compare with contralateral side or normal subject).

Nerve thickening is seen due to continuous frictional trauma (pressure injury), leprosy, hereditary neuropathies amyloidosis, and sarcoidosis.

- Also, feel for any neurofibromas along the course of nerves.
- Evaluate for *Tinel's sign* (distal paresthesia's along the nerve on tapping the nerve, e.g., at the site of injury or compression and regeneration.)

11.4 Neurocutaneous Markers

Phakomatosis refers to a group of neuro-oculo-cutaneous syndromes involving structures arising from the embryonic ectoderm. These disorders are characterized by lesions involving CNS, skin, and eyes. Evaluation of the patient for skin and eye abnormalities may provide a clue to the type of central nervous disorder.

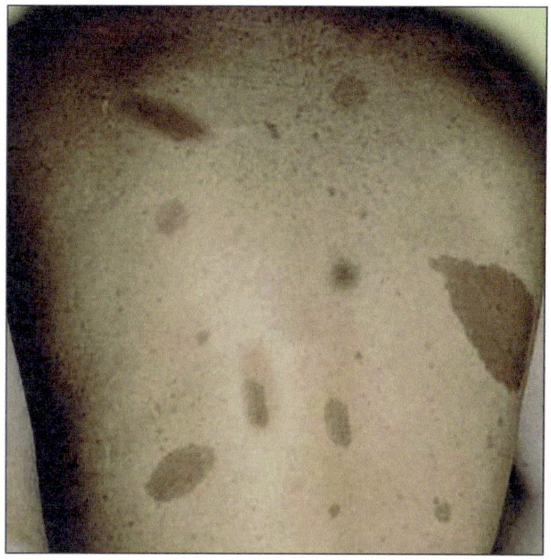

Fig. 11.5 Café-au-lait

11.4.1 Neurofibroma

Diagnosed by identifying six or more light brown (café au Lait spots) or at least two neurofibromas and at least one growth on the iris of eye or scoliosis.

- *NF 1* = café au lait spots and peripheral nerve neurofibromas
- *NF 2* = Bilateral acoustic neurofibromas with or without other CNS tumors (Fig. 11.5)

11.4.2 Sturge Weber Syndrome

Port wine stain on forehead, scalp, or around eye associated with glaucoma and leptomeningeal angiomas (Fig. 11.6).

11.4.3 Tuberous Sclerosis

Autosomal dominant disorder with lesions of skin and nonmalignant tumors in the brain and

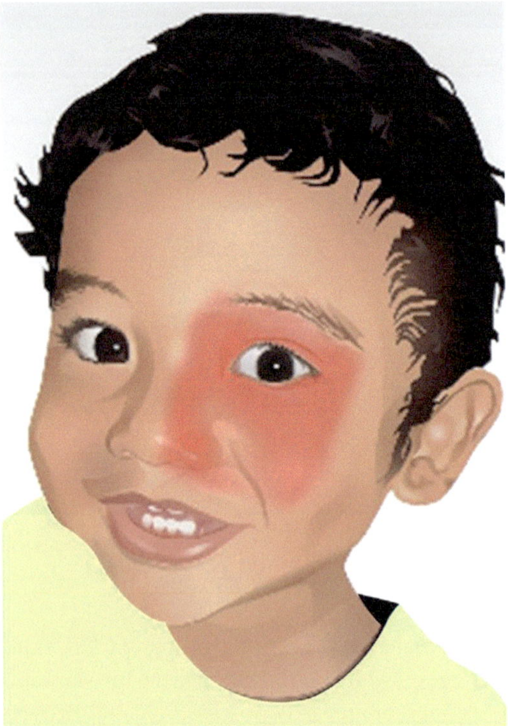

Fig. 11.6 Sturge Weber

other organs including kidney, liver, eyes, and lungs.

1. Skin—Hypomelanic macules (Ash leaf spots) seen better in UV light.
   (a) Facial angiofibroma's (reddish papules on nose and butterfly distribution)
   (b) Ungual fibromas
   (c) Shagreen patches (thick, orange peel-like pigmented and dimpled elevated lesions).
2. Retinal—Hamartomas
3. Pancreas—Neuroendocrine tumors
4. Kidneys—Angiomyolipoma
5. Lungs—Multiple cysts (lymphangioleiomyomatosis)
6. Cardiac—Rhabdomyomas (Fig. 11.7)

11.4.4 Ataxia telangiectasia

Autosomal recessive disorder with ataxia (cerebellar degeneration), oculomotor apraxia, and telangiectasia (dilated blood vessels) over sclera of both eyes (appear by 5–8 years of age) (Fig. 11.8).

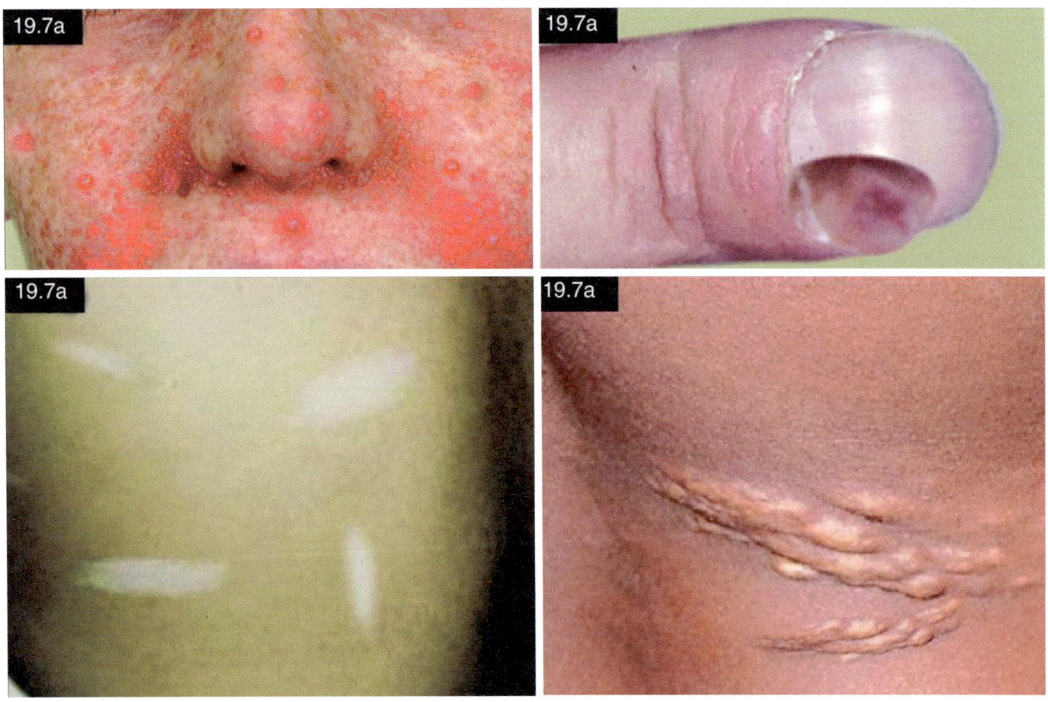

a. Adenoma sebacium
b. Periungual fibroma
c. Ash leaf hypopigmented patches
d. Shagreen patch

Fig. 11.7 Tuberous sclerosis (**a**–**d**)

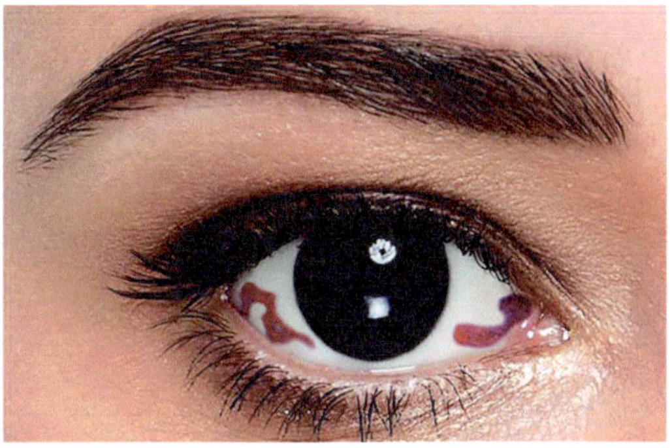

Fig. 11.8 Ataxia telangiectasia

11.4.5 Hypomelanosis of Ito

Streaked, whorled, or mottled patches of hypopigmentation in a segmental distribution, especially involving more than two body segments. Neurological findings include seizures, developmental delays, and scoliosis (Fig. 11.9).

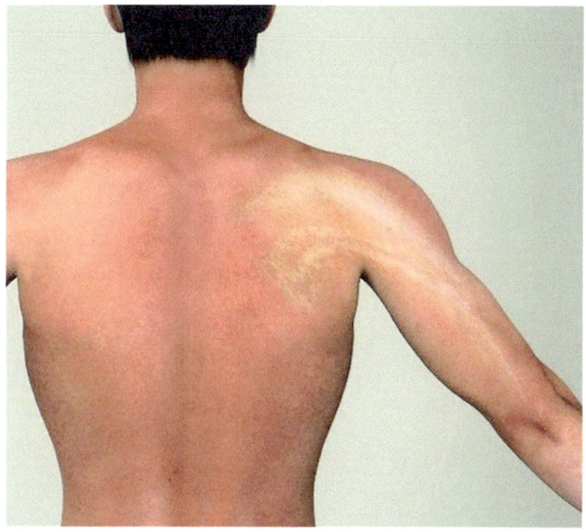

Fig. 11.9 Hypomelanosis of ito

11.4.6 Von-Hippel-Lindau Disease

Characterized by visceral cysts and benign tumors with subsequent potential for malignant transformation.

Patients have Angiomas (ocular), Hemangioblastomas, Pheochromocytomas, Renal cell carcinoma, pancreatic cysts, and detection of these tumors specific to the disease with a positive family history suggests the diagnosis.

12 Autonomic Nervous System Examination

Almost every organ from skin to glands to multiple viscera are supplied by the autonomic nervous system, which is divided into sympathetic and parasympathetic systems.

The *Sympathetic nervous system* is composed of noradrenergic, adrenergic, and cholinergic systems and neurons arises from multiple T1 to L2 thoracolumbar chain ganglia.

It acts as the "ALARM" system of the body and gets active in stressful situations to result in tachycardia, dilation of bronchi, inhibition of micturition (contraction of the internal urethral sphincter and relaxation of the detrusor), increased sweating, mydriasis, and reduced bowel motility (Fig. 12.1).

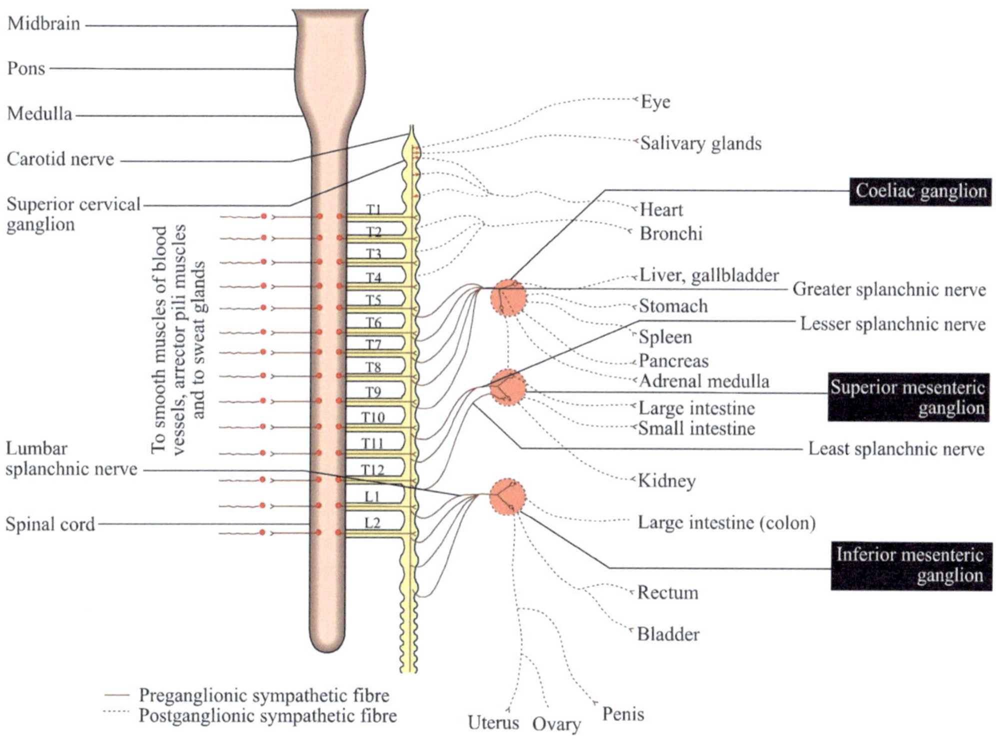

Fig. 12.1 Sympathetic pathway

V. Suri, *Clinical Neurological Examination and Localization*,
https://doi.org/10.1007/978-981-16-1228-2_12

The *Parasympathetic nervous system* is composed of cholinergic neurons and arise from the brainstem cranial nuclei (3rd, 7th, 9th, 10th nuclei) or sacral spinal cord (S2–S4).

It acts as the "RELAX" system of the body resulting in bradycardia, bronchial constriction, Initiation of micturition (contraction of detrusor and relaxation of the internal urethral sphincter), erection, constriction of the pupil, and increased salivation and lacrimation (Fig. 12.2).

The history and physical examination of the autonomic nervous system should be performed keeping certain important key points in mind.

Autonomic nervous system	Symptoms and signs
Sympathetic noradrenergic system	
• Failure • Hyperactivity	• Orthostatic hypotension • Palpitations, elevated BP pupillary dilatation, piloerection, and skin pallor
Sympathetic adrenergic system	
• Failure • Hyperactivity	• Fatigue—nonspecific • Palpitations, pallor, dilated pupil
Sympathetic cholinergic system	
• Failure • Hyperactivity	• Hypohidrosis with resultant heat intolerance • Hyperhidrosis—focal, e.g., palms and soles or generalized
Parasympathetic cholinergic system	
• Failure – Cranial component – Sacral component • Hyperactivity	• Decreased salivation and tearing, pupillary dilatation, constipation • Urinary retention • Erectile dysfunction • Increased salivation and lacrimation, slow heart rate, increased urine frequency, and urgency

12.1 History

History should include certain important symptoms, which may provide a clue to the site of lesion.

- Urinary—hesitancy, urgency, incontinence, bladder sensation-evaluate for both voiding and holding symptoms
- Stool—constipation, incontinence
- Sweating—abnormal (hypohidrosis or hyperhidrosis), region of abnormality (focal or generalized)
- Salivation and lacrimation—reduced or increased
- Heart rate and blood pressure—elevated or reduced
- Erectile dysfunction, ejaculatory dysfunction
- Postural hypotension with related postural dizziness, light-headed feeling, and syncopal feeling.

12.2 Tests for Autonomic Nervous System

12.2.1 Inspection of skin

Sympathetic lesion:

1. Flushing of skin
2. Warmth of Skin
3. Sweating absent in sympathetic cholinergic lesion with excessive sweating in hyperactivity.

12.2.2 Cardiovascular Reflexes

These tests are based on the response of the sympathetic (noradrenergic and adrenergic) and parasympathetic nerve supply of the heart and blood vessels.

1. *Postural hypotension*
   (a) Occurs in patients with failure of sympathetic noradrenergic system.
   (b) Patient should initially lie supine and rested for 2 min and then is asked to stand. Healthy persons may also have an initial drop of BP during the first 20–30 s of standing and hence BP measurement for orthostatic hypotension should be done after standing for at least 1 min.
   (c) Orthostatic hypotension is defined by BP drop of >30 mm systolic or >15 mm diastolic in upright posture. Orthostatic hypotension is defined only by the drop of Bp and not only by postural symptoms.
2. *BP response to*
   (a) Mental arithmetic

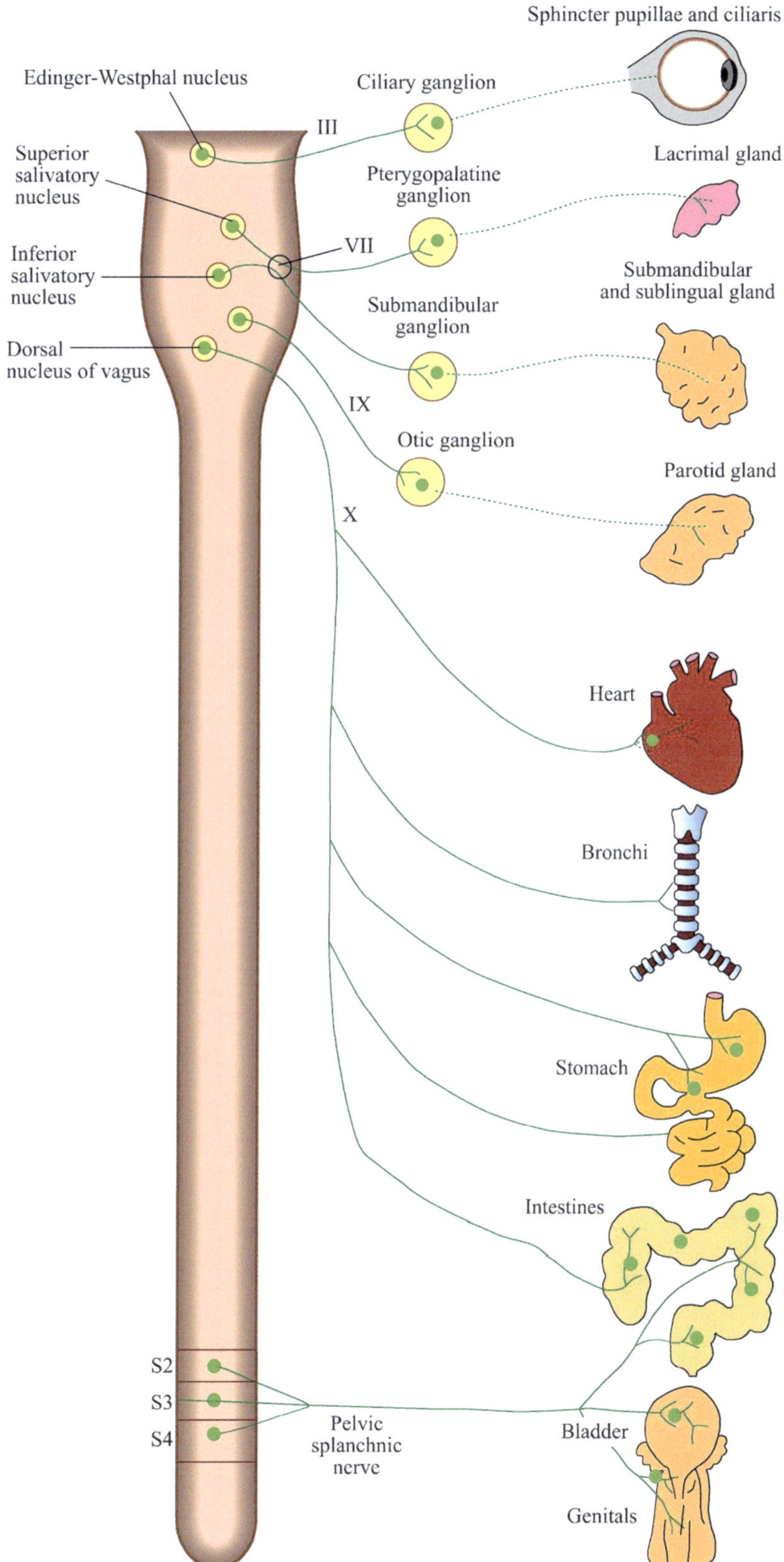

Fig 12.2 Cerebro-sacral parasympathetic pathway

   (b) Sustained handgrip
   (c) Exposure to cold

   Diastolic BP should rise with these activities by >10 mm. Abnormal response (<10 mm BP elevation) is seen in sympathetic lesions.
3. *Heart rate response or Cardiovagal tests*
   (a) The parasympathetic influence by the vagus nerve on the heart rate is assessed by various activities including deep breathing, valsalva, and change of posture.
   (b) Continuous ECG on a single lead ECG tracing is obtained (rhythm strip) and variation in RR interval is assessed in response to various activities.

E:I Ratio

ECG is recorded in *deep* inspiration and expiration at a frequency of 6 breaths/min. Compare the longest RR to the shortest RR.

- Normal > 1.2.
- Abnormal response in parasympathetic dysfunction.

30:15 Beat Ratio

ECG is recorded in lying down and then patient is made to stand. Compare the RR ratio post standing of beat 15 to beat 30.

- normal > 1.04
- Abnormal response (no change) seen in parasympathetic lesion.

Valsalva Ratio

The recumbent patient is asked to exhale against a closed glottis or against a manometer to maintain the mercury level at 30–40 mm mercury for 15 s.

Variation of shortest to longest RR is compared during and post Valsalva.

- normal > 1.21
- Abnormal response in parasympathetic dysfunction

12.2.3 Sweating Tests or Sudomotor Tests

1. Skin is dried and then dusted with quinizarin powder. Patient is placed in a heat cradle or near a warming device and given a hot drink with 500 mg paracetamol. Areas of sweating are outlined as the powder turns black in areas of sweating.
   (a) Abnormal—sympathetic cholinergic dysfunction—loss of sweating in segment distribution, or below a spinal level or in different body parts.
2. QSART (quantitative sudomotor axon reflex test) Iontophoresis of acetylcholine at the skin surface activates an axon reflex that travels antidromically to a branch point in the peripheral nerve and then orthodromically to evoke a sudomotor response in the nearby eccrine glands leading to production of sweat. The response is measured by the amount of moisture produced and detected over a certain time by collection in a capsule placed over the skin. It is an important test for the detection of small fiber dysfunction.
3. Skin Sympathetic Response (SSR)

   Surface electrodes over hand or foot are used and recording is conducted after electrical stimulation. Skin sympathetic response (SSR) is a slow wave resulting from activation of the sudomotor sympathetic efferent fibers. SSR is considered abnormal if no significant response is elicited. SSR is a simple and reliable indicator of sympathetic sudomotor outflow in central and peripheral nervous disorders.

12.2.4 Rectum

LMN Lesion

- Incontinence
- Absence of anal reflex and lax internal anal sphincter on the gloved finger.

UMN Lesion

- Constipation
- Maintained internal anal sphincter contractions on gloved finger.

12.2.5 Bladder

- Sensation of bladder is normally felt at 100–150 ml urine.
- Rhythmic detrusor contraction with a slight desire to pass urine starts at 400–600 ml.

UMN bladder (lesions from Frontal lobe till cord above S2, S3, S4) results in a spastic, low capacity bladder.

LMN bladder involving local arc at S2, S3, S4 results in a hypotonic bladder with reduced sensation, reduced contraction, high residual urine, and overflow incontinence.

Bladder pressure and urodynamics should be evaluated by micturition cystometrogram and uroflowmetry.

12.2.6 Pupillary Signs

Pupil is examined in a darkened room with the patient gazing into the distance.

Sympathetic deficit—reduces pupil size and is more apparent in dim light. Horner's syndrome results in ptosis, miosis, facial anhidrosis, enophthalmos, and loss of ciliospinal reflex.

Parasympathetic deficit—causes an enlarged and tonic pupil.

12.2.7 Laboratory Tests

Certain laboratory tests are conducted for various autonomic disorders.

- Plasma metanephrine level—phaechromocytoma
- 24-h urine hydroxyindoleacetic acid—carcinoid syndrome
- plasma histamine level—mast cell degranulation disorder

Test	Normal/abnormal	Dysfunction Parasympathetic/ sympathetic
1. Skin	• Abnormal warmth and flushing	Sympathetic
	• Abnormal sweating	Sympathetic cholinergic
2. Cardiovascular reflexes		
(a) Postural hypotension	BP drop >30/15	Sympathetic noradrenergic
(b) BP response to mental arithmetic, sustained handgrip, exposure to cold	Abnormal if diastolic rise <10 mm	Sympathetic adrenergic lesion
(c) Heart rate response		
E:I	Abnormal < 1.2	Parasympathetic defect
30:15 best ratio	Abnormal < 1.04	Parasympathetic defect
Valsalva ratio	Abnormal < 1.21	Parasympathetic defect
3. Sweating test	Loss or absence of sweating or hyperhidrosis	Sympathetic cholinergic defect
4. Skin sympathetic response (SSR)	Slow wave resulting from activation of sudomotor sympathetic efferent fibers	Sympathetic defect

13 Examination of the Unconscious Patient

Evaluation of the unconscious or poorly responsive. patient requires an organized and focused approach that need not take a long time if the examination is focused and organized.

Three important questions need to be answered when examining an unconscious patient:

1. What is the level of consciousness?
2. Is the neurological examination focal or generalized?
3. What is the possible site and etiology of the neurological problem?

13.1 Q 1. What Is the Level of Consciousness?

Coma is defined as a deep state of unconsciousness from which the patient cannot be awakened and cannot respond purposefully to environmental stimulation.

1. The most common method to describe the state of unconsciousness and which is most popular amongst neurologists is to *describe the EXACT STATE of the patient* in terms of what the patient can do and what the patient cannot do, e.g., "patient is drowsy, arousable to deep pain to transiently open eyes and fixate gaze but cannot obey verbal commands and has a reduced attention span." This is preferred over the specific scales like the Glasgow coma scale, which is a scale more specific for head injured patients and evaluates the "best response" rather than the "worst response." Hence a patient with stroke may have worsening motor responses on the hemiplegic side but the best response that is rated for the GCS may not drop.

   Certain commonly used terms by neurologists to describe the level of consciousness are described here though their specific description may not be precisely similar with different neurologists. In increasing order of worsening of the level of consciousness these include:

(a) *Lethargic patient*

   Patient is dull though arousable but has reduced wakefulness and awareness and has reduced attention span with impaired orientation.

(b) *Obtunded patient*

   Patient is somnolent and shows little or no interest in the surroundings and is bradyphrenic (paucity of thoughts) on being aroused.

(c) *Stupor*

   Has only minimal response to maximal painful response and only a vigorous stimulus can transiently arouse the patient who does not perform any significant response and returns promptly to unresponsive state

V. Suri, *Clinical Neurological Examination and Localization*,
https://doi.org/10.1007/978-981-16-1228-2_13

(d) *Coma*

Patient is unarousable with closed eyes even to deep painful and vigorous stimulation

2. *Glasgow coma scale*

Provides a more replicable and objective description of the neurological status of the unconscious patient. The best *E*ye (E), best *V*erbal (V), and best *M*otor (M) response are recorded. The lowest score possible, suggestive of deep coma is 3 and the best score suggestive of normal consciousness is 15.

	1	2	3	4	5	6
Eye (E) 4	Does not open	Opens to pain	Opens to voice	Opens spontaneously		
Verbal (V) 5	Makes no sound	Makes sound	Speaks words	Confused and disoriented	Oriented	
Motor (M) 6	No movement	Extension to pain	Abnormal flexion to pain	Flexion to pain	Localizes pain	Obeys commands

Locked in State

Patient is mute, motionless, unable to produce motor response except eye blinking, or ocular movements. Patient is, however, awake and aware of self and is capable of perceiving sensory stimulation. Seen in brainstem lesions, Guillaine barre syndrome.

Akinetic Mutism

Patient appears awake but has "paucity of thought, action, and speech" though with normal language and corticospinal tract function. Seen in patients with bilateral frontal lobe dysfunction.

Vegetative State

Patient has a lack of awareness of self and environment with lack of ability to perceive or respond to external stimuli though they have preserved vital vegetative functions, e.g., maintenance of blood pressure with preserved sleep–wake cycle. They are incontinent. The vegetative state that persists for more than 3 months is labeled as *persistent vegetative state* and these patients are unlikely to have any significant further neurological recovery.

Minimal Conscious State

Patient has severely altered consciousness but unlike vegetative state these patients have minimal but definite evidence of self or environmental awareness. These patients may respond minimally and inconsistently to some simple commands, e.g., moving a finger or blinking the eye to external stimuli.

13.2 Q 2. Is the Neurological Examination Focal or Generalized?

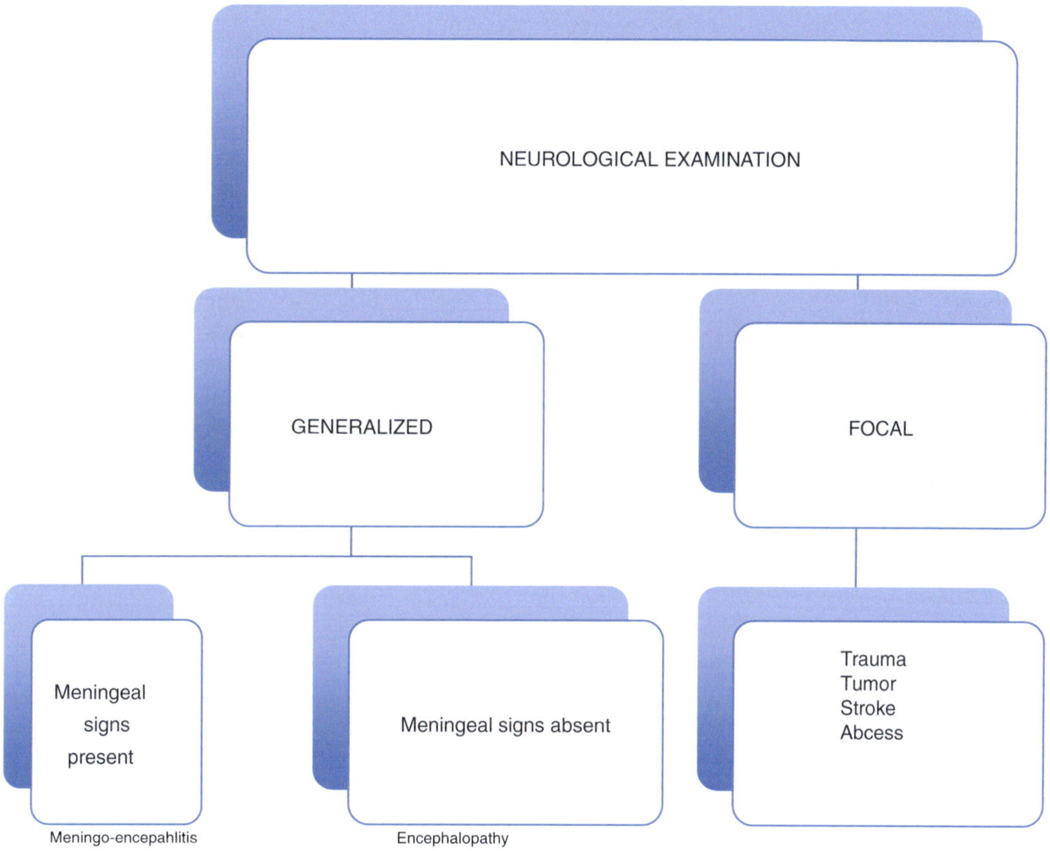

Soft or definite focal neurological signs may indicate a focal loss of function in the nervous system indicative of focal structural lesion, e.g., tumors, stroke, and trauma. These patients have to be differentiated from patients who do not have a focal neurological deficit and these patients with a generalized neurological examination are likely to have encephalopathies or meningoencephalitis.

Signs which are suggestive of a possibility of a focal lesion include:

- Asymmetry of facial grimace with poor naso-labial fold and wider palpebral fissure on one side.
- Asymmetrical movement of limbs in response to deep central or peripheral pain. Limbs may also show asymmetrical tone and different speeds of fall from an elevated position.
- Conjugate gaze palsies, skew deviation.
- Asymmetrical reflexes (deep tendon reflexes) and unilateral extensor plantar response.

Patients who have focal deficits are more likely to have a focal CNS lesion, e.g., stroke, trauma, tumor, or abscess.

Patients with a non-focal CNS examination should be evaluated for the presence or absence of *meningeal signs*. A non-focal CNS examination with meningeal signs is suggestive of meningoencephalitis. A non-focal CNS examination without any meningeal signs is suggestive of an encephalopathy (toxic, metabolic, or alternate).

Meningeal Signs

1. *Nuchal rigidity*—difficulty and restriction of forward neck flexion with normal side to side neck movement.
2. *Kernig's sign*—thigh is flexed at the hip and at the knee to 90* angle and then gradually the knee is extended. Resistance to knee extension due to pain and resistance from the muscles with stiffness of the muscles is considered as suggestive of meningismus (Fig. 13.1).
3. *Brudzinski's sign*—forced forward flexion of the neck results in reflex flexion of hips and upper limbs and also indicates presence of meningismus (Fig. 13.2).

13.3 Q3 What Is the Possible Site and Etiology of the Lesion?

This is the most important part of the examination of the unconscious patient and certain localizing features are observed on the patient.

13.3.1 Pattern of Respiration (Fig. 13.3)

(a) *Cheyne's stoke respiration*

Cheyne—stoke respiration is characterized by progressively increasing and deeper respiration with increasing rate followed by gradual decrease in rate and amplitude of respiration followed by a phase of apnea occurring in a crescendo–decrescendo fashion.

It indicates preserved brain stem function and may be seen in metabolic encephalopathies, diencephalic lesion, raised intracranial pressure, or diffuse cortical dysfunction.

(b) *Central neurogenic hyperventilation*

Patients have deep and rapid rates of breathing usually with rates of >25/min with

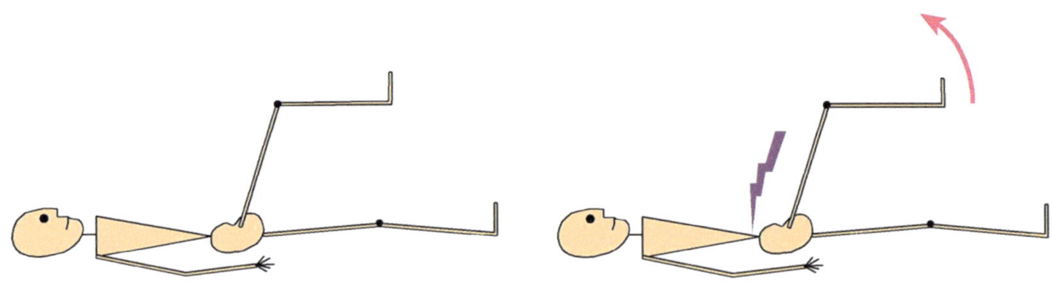

Fig. 13.1 Kernig's sign

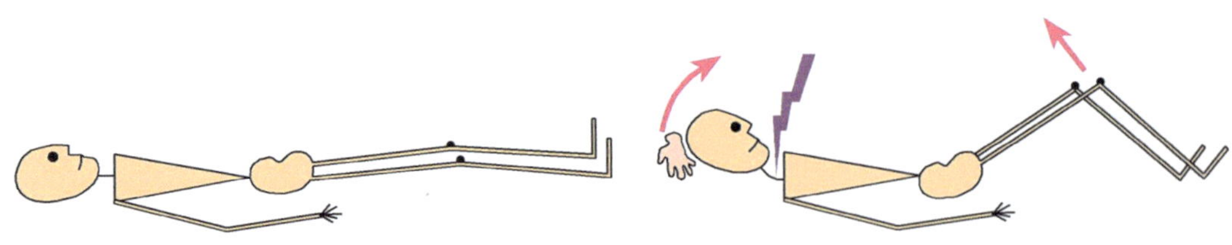

Fig. 13.2 Brudzinski's sign

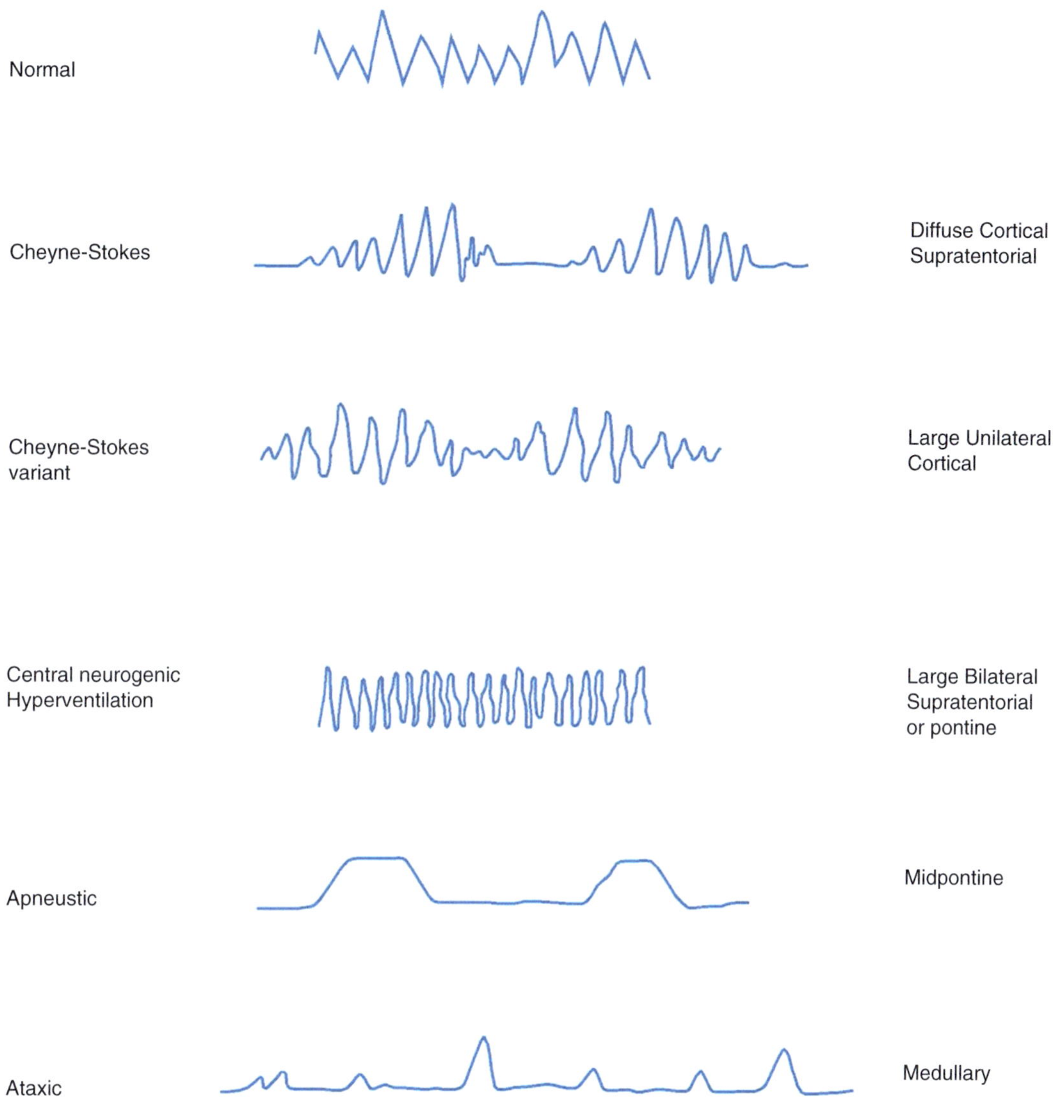

Fig. 13.3 Patterns of respiration

resultant increase in PaO_2, decreased $PaCO_2$, and increased pH. Maybe seen in patients with dysfunction of large bilateral cortical or pons and medullary dysfunction.

(c) *Apneustic breathing*

Patients have a 2–3 s phase of apnea following full inspiration. This pattern of breathing is seen in patients with Pontine dysfunction.

(d) *Ataxia or Bitot breathing*

Also called gasping or agonal breathing and is seen in patients with medullary dysfunction.

Breathing is gasping with irregular patterns and variable strength of each breath with irregular gap between each breath.

13.3.2 Motor Status

1. *Hemiplegic posturing*—reduced facial movement, reduced unilateral arm and leg movement, unilateral extensor plantar may indicate a focal lesion in the contralateral cerebral hemisphere or ipsilateral brain stem (Fig. 13.4).

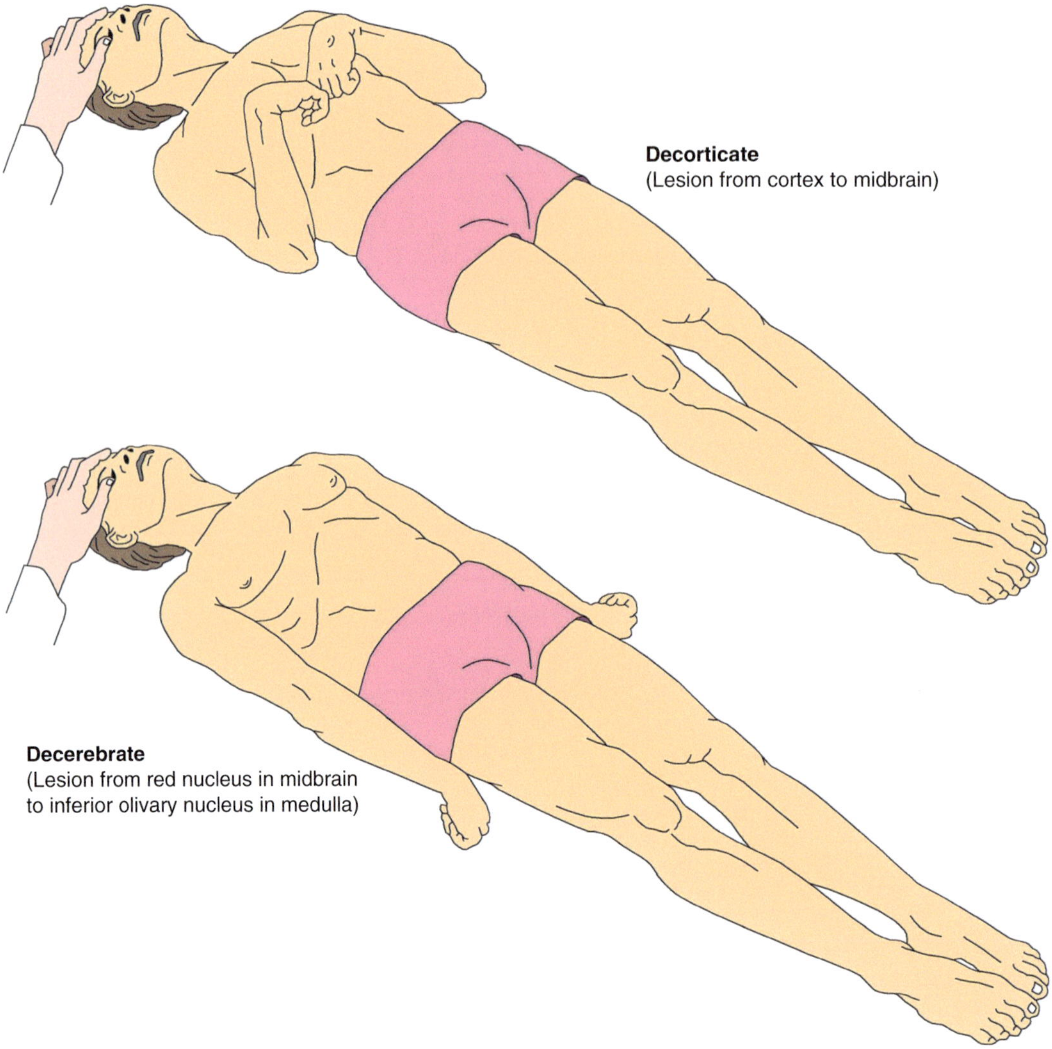

Fig. 13.4 Decorticate and decerebrate posturing

2. *Decorticate posturing*
   (a) Patient has generalized stiffness with flexed elbows and wrists and clenched fists with hyperextended legs.
   (b) Caused by damage to corticospinal tract or rubrospinal tract from cortex up to red nucleus in the midbrain, e.g., cortex, internal capsule, thalamus, midbrain above red nucleus (to remember—de CORTICAte, i.e., loss of cortical input to red nucleus and lesion proximal to red nucleus).
3. *Decerebrate posturing*
   (a) Patient has a state of generalized stiffness with adducted and extended arms, especially at elbows with pronation of forearm and hyperextension of legs with plantar flexion of ankles.
   (b) Caused by lesion of brainstem occurring from the red nucleus in the midbrain to the inferior olivary nucleus in the medulla.

13.3.3 Pupils

Observe for anisocoria (asymmetry of pupil size is significant if the difference on both sides is >0.5 mm)

- Diencephalic lesion or metabolic encephalopathy—2–3 mm reactive pupils
- Midbrain lesion—4–5 mm, irregular and non-reactive pupil
- Pontine lesions—pin point and reactive pupils
- Medullary lesion—Horner's syndrome
- Uncal herniation—Ipsilateral nonreactive pupil with 3rd-nerve palsy and contralateral extensor plantar (Kernohan sign)

13.3.4 Ocular Movements

Evaluate for conjugate horizontal or vertical gaze palsies or gaze preference.

Evaluate ocular movements by eliciting the doll's eye or oculo-cephalic response where horizontal and vertical (forward flexion or hyperextension) head movement should result in complete and symmetrical conjugate movement to the opposite side.

Conjugate Deviation Conjugate palsy to the right maybe seen in lesions of left frontal eye field area up to the oculomotor decussation or of the right-sided PPRF.

Disconjugate Gaze For example, isolated ocular adduction failure and intact vertical movements may indicate a lesion of MLF.

Skew Deviation Vertical misalignment of the eyes. Occurs due to supranuclear lesions from brain to oculomotor nuclei. The hypotropic or lower-placed eye usually corresponds to the side of lesion.

Upgaze or Downgaze Palsy Seen in lesions of rostral interstitial nucleus of medial longitudinal fasciculus (ri MLF) or lesion of interstitial nucleus of Cajal or the posterior commissure.

Ocular Bobbing Fast downward movement of patient's eye and usually seen in pontine lesions (Fig. 13.5).

13.3.5 Reflexes

Evaluate for asymmetry of superficial and deep tendon reflexes and plantar responses, which may indicate the site of lesion by providing a reflex level.

13.3.6 Sensory Evaluation

Marginally obtunded and intubated patients may be aroused to cooperate for assessment of pain, temperature, touch, or vibration sensations where the patient may be able to respond by gestures.

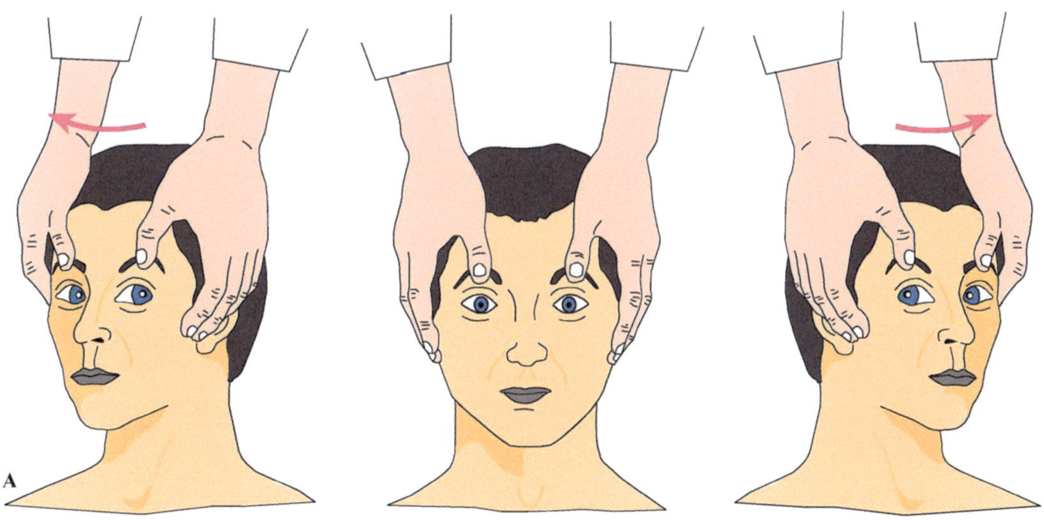

Fig. 13.5 Vestibulo-ocular reflex

In comatosed patients response to deep pain on either side maybe assessed by the motor response to pain and loss of pain sensations on one limb or one half of the body would provide a clue to a focal CNS examination.

13.3.7 Other Aspects of Neurological Evaluation

1. Skull examination
   (a) Injuries may be hidden below the hair
   (b) Burr holes indicative of old surgeries
   (c) Any bony deformity suggesting an exostosis tumor
2. Signs of meningeal irritation
   (a) Neck rigidity—assess for resistance to flexion and extension of the neck. Resistance in all neck movements including lateral movements as well may indicate spondylotic or ankylosing disease of the cervical spine.
   (b) Kernigs sign—the thigh is flexed at the hip and knee is kept at 90°. Kernig's test is considered positive and indicates meningeal irritation if a further extension of the knee is both painful and leads to resistance to the movement.
   (c) Brudizinski's sign—is positive and indicates meningeal irritation when passive forward flexion of the neck leads to raising up the knees and hips in flexion.
3. Ear examination
   (a) Tenderness over the mastoid may indicate mastoiditis and may point toward an intracranial infection from the middle ear.
   (b) Bleeding from the ear may indicate a base of skull fracture.
   (c) Battle's sign or mastoid ecchymosis (extravasation of blood along the path of posterior auricular artery) may indicate a fracture of the middle cranial fossa.
4. Tongue examination
   (a) Bilateral lateral tongue bites strongly indicate a generalized seizure.
   (b) Abnormal discoloration or corrosive effect on the tongue may indicate poisoning.
5. Fundus examination
   (a) Presence of papilledema indicates raised intracranial pressure.
   (b) It must be remembered that papilledema may be absent in a number of space-occupying lesions, especially when they have evolved rapidly. Absence of papilledema hence does not exclude raised intracranial pressure though its presence is indicative of raised intracranial pressure.

14 Summary of Localization

14.1 LMN Lesions

1. Hypotonia
2. Prominent wasting
3. Absent superficial and deep tendon reflexes
4. Plantar response flexor

Anterior horn cell	Pure motor
	Marked wasting
	Prominent fasciculations
Root	Pure motor or pure sensory deficit in preganglionic and sensori-motor in postganglionic involvement
	Root or dermatomal distribution of deficit
	Root pain common
Plexus	Mixed motor and sensory deficit
	Multiple contiguous nerves involved
Nerve	1. Mononeuropathy—single nerve
	2. Mononeuritis multiplex—multifocal noncontiguous nerves involved
	3. Polyneuropathy—length dependent involvement—short glove and long stocking distribution of sensory and motor deficit

Neuromuscular junction	Muscle
1. Pure motor	1. Pure motor
2. True fatiguability observed	2. Select group of muscles involved e.g., proximal, facioscapulohumoral
3. Select group of muscles involved	3. Pseudohypertrophy of muscles
	4. DTR loss is proportionate to motor power.

14.2 UMN Lesion and Sites

1. Spasticity (clasp knife)
2. Loss of superficial reflexes
3. Brisk deep tendon reflexes
4. Plantar extensor
5. No or minimal wasting

Cortex	1. Non-dense contralateral hemiplegia
	2. Seizures
	3. Cortical signs, e.g., agnosia, apraxia, cortical sensory loss
Corona radiata	1. Non-dense contralateral hemiplegia
	2. Absent cortical signs
Internal capsule	1. Dense contralateral hemiplegia
	2. Contralateral Hemisensory deficit
	3. Ataxic hemiparesis (pyramidal and cerebellar signs on same side but contralateral to lesion)

V. Suri, *Clinical Neurological Examination and Localization*,
https://doi.org/10.1007/978-981-16-1228-2_14

Thalamus	1. Subtle contralateral hemiparesis
	2. Hemisensory contralateral deficit
	3. Contralateral ataxic hemiparesis
Midbrain	1. Contralateral hemiplegia
	2. Ipsilateral 3rd or 4th cranial palsy
Pons	1. Contralateral hemiplegia
	2. Ipsilateral 5th, 6th, 7th palsy
Medulla	1. Lateral—ipsilateral 5th (trigeminal tract), 9th, 10th, cerebellar and contralateral pain and temperature loss.
	2. Anterior—contralateral hemiplegia with ipsilateral 12th
Cord	1. Partial—Brown Sequard syndrome
	Contralateral hemiplegia/monoplegia of leg, with extensor plantar
	Contralateral pain and temperature loss
	Ipsilateral light touch, vibration, and joint position loss
	Ipsilateral autonomic dystonia
	2. Complete cord syndrome resulting in deficit below the involved spinal segment. Flexor spasms indicate complete cord involvement with involvement of Reticulo-spinal and Tectospinal tracts
	Extradural involvement - Local bony pain at site of lesion, local bony deformity or tenderness, Symmetrical onset deficit, root pain at site of lesion in 90% of patients. Clinical prototype - spondylosis, Potts spine, Extradural bone metastasis
	Intradural involvement - Absence of local pain, deformity, Root pains at level of lesion in 100%, Asymetrical onset of deficit which may later become symmetrical. Prototype - Neurofibroma, Meningioma
	Intramedullary involvement - Dissociate anaesthesia (involvement of pain and temperature with preserved light touch) in suspended distribution, early bladder and bowel involvement, rapid progression to invole multiple long tracts. Prototype - Myelitis, tumors of cord, syrinx.

MIX
Papier aus verantwortungsvollen Quellen
Paper from responsible sources
FSC® C105338

If you have any concerns about our products,
you can contact us on
ProductSafety@springernature.com

In case Publisher is established outside the EU,
the EU authorized representative is:
Springer Nature Customer Service Center GmbH
Europaplatz 3, 69115 Heidelberg, Germany

Printed by Libri Plureos GmbH
in Hamburg, Germany